The Occasional Human Sacrifice

THE OCCASIONAL HUMAN SACRIFICE

Medical Experimentation and the Price of Saying No

CARL ELLIOTT

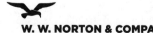

W. W. NORTON & COMPANY

Independent Publishers Since 1923

For information about permission to reproduce selections from this book, write to
Permissions, W. W. Norton & Company, Inc., 500 Fifth Avenue, New York, NY 10110

For information about special discounts for bulk purchases, please contact
W. W. Norton Special Sales at specialsales@wwnorton.com or 800-233-4830

Manufacturing by Lakeside Book Company
Book design by Lisa Buckley
Production manager: Gwen Cullen

ISBN 978-1-324-06550-0

W. W. Norton & Company, Inc., 500 Fifth Avenue, New York, N.Y. 10110
www.wwnorton.com

W. W. Norton & Company Ltd., 15 Carlisle Street, London W1D 3BS

1 2 3 4 5 6 7 8 9 0

To Leigh Turner

Every whistleblower is an amateur playing against professionals.

—JOHN PESANDO

Contents

The Occasional Human Sacrifice

Introduction

L et me present my credentials as a coward. Picture me at age twenty-four, a third-year medical student, clean-shaven and dressed in a short white coat, like a barber. I have just started an internal medicine rotation at the VA hospital in Charleston, South Carolina, where I have been told to perform a bone marrow biopsy. Have I ever performed a bone marrow biopsy before? No. Do I know how to perform a bone marrow biopsy? Again, no. But it is understood that medical students should "be aggressive," especially when it comes to invasive procedures. I should want to do a bone marrow biopsy. I should be fighting my way to the front of the line, shoving and elbowing the other students aside. "See one, do one, teach one" is the cardinal rule of medical training, and while the details are hazy, I have seen a bone marrow biopsy before. "Just pretend you know what you're doing," I tell myself, my forehead shining with sweat.

A bone marrow biopsy is not an enormously complicated procedure. It typically involves inserting a long, hollow needle into the patient's pelvic bone in order to extract a sample of bone marrow. But it can be very painful, especially in the trembling, unskilled hands of a medical student. My friend Scott Campbell underwent a bone marrow biopsy once when he got lymphoma in the 1990s. His procedure was performed by an experienced physician, and Scott claims it was easily the worst pain he has ever experienced, ranking it over a ruptured appendix, a torn meniscus, a shard of metal in his eye, a ruptured vertebral disk, and chemotherapy.

I would like to report that I was brave enough to back out of doing this procedure without help. I would like to say that I didn't deliver a gruesome serving of pain to an elderly Black veteran, lying on his side as I struggled to twist a large-bore metal needle into his iliac crest. I would like to claim that the procedure didn't take an exceptionally long period of time, one made even longer by the groans and shudders of my victim. But that would not be true. Like the subjects in Stanley Milgram's obedience experiments, I did as I was told. I pretended I knew what I was doing. The possibility of objecting never occurred to me.

Nor did I object when I was told to perform lumbar punctures, episiotomies, arterial sticks, or any number of other invasive procedures without proper supervision. More than once on my gynecology rotation I was invited by an attending to feel the cervix of an anesthetized woman lying on the operating table. Had she given consent to have a group of medical students perform a pelvic exam on her while she was unconscious? Did she have any idea that when the lights went out she would become a clinical practice dummy, her genitals palpated by a series of gloved hands? Probably not. I never asked. I just did as I was told.

When I was rotating through consult-liaison psychiatry, a young man was admitted to the intensive care unit, paralyzed from the neck down as the result of a diving accident. Another medical student and I listened as the psychiatry resident interviewed him. The patient, barely out of high school, was devastated by his injury. The future he had envisioned for himself had vanished with a crack of his spinal column, and in its place, he could see nothing but dependence and loneliness. Tears were streaming down his face. After a short silence, the resident asked him, "Have you thought about getting a trained monkey?" As my fellow medical student and I looked at each other in stunned disbelief, the resident proceeded to tell the paralyzed patient about the remarkable array of household tasks that monkeys could be trained to perform. There was no need to be depressed! The future was bright! How did I respond to this bizarre speech? Did I object, interrupt, or apologize to the patient? No, I did not. I stared at the floor in silence.

Should I continue? When I rotated through internal medicine at the county hospital, our team needed to put a central line in an older Black man who was still groggy from anesthesia. A nurse objected that the man was unable to consent and asked the resident to wait until he was clearheaded. But the senior resident was a very busy man. He didn't want to wait. After fuming and pacing for a few minutes, he came up with a plan: Give the patient naloxone—Narcan—to reverse the effects of anesthesia. "Wait a second," one of the interns said. "This guy is groggy from a benzo. Does naloxone reverse the effects of benzodiazepines?" The senior resident started laughing. "No, of course not. But the nurse doesn't know that." In went a bolus of IV naloxone, and out came the consent form for the dazed old man to sign. Did I know this was wrong? Yes. Did I object? No, I did not.

I could go on. The case file on my cowardice is large. It extends well beyond my time in medical school. But my intention isn't to confess my sins. I just want to emphasize that it is not in my nature to be confrontational. I don't send back food in restaurants. I don't shush people in theaters. I don't honk my horn in traffic. I didn't march in protests in college or construct anti-apartheid shantytowns on the lawn next to the president's house. For years I was so nervous about giving public lectures that I had to take beta-blockers to keep my voice from quavering. For most of my life I have been the son who obeyed his parents, the player who obeyed the coach, the medical student who obeyed the attendings. All of which makes it hard to explain why I launched an all-consuming, self-destructive, seven-year public crusade against my own employer on behalf of a mistreated research subject who was already dead.

This is a book about whistleblowers, not a book about me. It was not my intention to write about the suicide of Dan Markingson at the University of Minnesota or my struggle to have his death investigated. But it would be disingenuous to pretend that my interest in whistleblowing did not come out of that experience or that it had no effect on the way I have written this book. I have spent the past several years in the company of whistleblowers, trying to understand their stories, comparing each one to the others, attempting to see patterns and draw out common moral threads. I hope that my own experience made me a more perceptive listener. But the opposite could be true, of course. It is possible that my experience has compromised my objectivity.

Although I graduated from medical school in 1987, I have never actually practiced medicine. Instead of starting a residency, I moved to Scotland to study philosophy. I have spent most of my life since then as a university professor. While the reasons behind that decision are complicated, a summary version would be something like this: Medical training was turning me into a terrible human being. I was becoming harder, meaner, and more entitled. The transformation wasn't complete; I was still able to step back, reflect on my actions, and feel bad about myself. But I could see what lay ahead.

Popular culture presents us with two different portraits of the whistleblower, each with a different moral valence. The first portrait is familiar from Hollywood movies: the brave, conscience-driven hero who risks everything to expose corruption and injustice. This portrait emphasizes the whistleblower's moral courage. The second portrait is more familiar from tabloid newspapers and television news reports: the aggrieved, disgruntled malcontent who snitches on the organization to settle a grudge. This portrait emphasizes the whistleblower's antisocial tendencies and willingness to make enemies. These portraits differ in their moral assessments, yet both reassure potential witnesses to wrongdoing that blowing the whistle is not something that normal people do.

Unless I squint hard, it is difficult for me to recognize myself in either of these portraits. In fact, it's not easy to recognize any actual human being in these portraits, including those I have written about in this book. The problem is not just that the pictures are caricatures, or that they are too simple, or even their assumption that whistleblowers are very unusual people. It is the idea that whistleblowers are fundamentally alike. This is not to deny that blowing the whistle demands principled dissent or that dissent can be very difficult. But if you were to meet the whistleblowers in this book without knowing their histories, it would be hard to see what they have in common. What they share is not a character trait but a common experience, and even that has turned out very differently for each of them.

How the experience turns out will color the story a whistleblower tells: what they remember, what they see as significant, how they judge themselves and the actions they took. It will also affect what they hear in the stories told by other whistleblowers. I can testify to this from firsthand experience. The book that you are reading is not the book I would have written fifteen years ago. It comes out of a moral sensibility that has been shaped by the experience of a particular event. Anyone reading a book about an ethical issue must decide whether they can trust the narrator. I want to be as honest as possible about where I stand.

• • •

Here is how I first learned about the death of Dan Markingson. My family and I were in an apartment complex near Camps Bay Beach, just outside of Cape Town, South Africa. It was June of 2008, and I was just finishing a year-long sabbatical from the University of Minnesota, where I worked as a professor in the Center for Bioethics. Into my email inbox one evening came a message from Paul Tosto, a reporter I was friendly with back in the Twin Cities. Paul wanted to get my opinion about a series he and a colleague, Jeremy Olson, had published in the *St. Paul Pioneer Press*.[1] The wireless signal in our apartment was weak, and I can remember walking around the courtyard of the complex in the dark, holding my laptop over my head, trying to find a spot where the signal was strong enough for me to read the articles.

The story Paul sent was deeply unsettling. On May 8, 2003, a young, mentally ill research subject named Dan Markingson had laid down in the bathtub of a halfway house and slashed his throat with a box cutter. His mutilated body was found in the early hours of the morning, along with a note that said, "I went through this experience smiling!" Stephen Olson, a psychiatrist at the University of Minnesota, had enrolled Markingson in a drug study over the objections of his mother, Mary Weiss, who had watched her son's mental state deteriorate for months. She had desperately tried to get him out of the study, but her pleas were ignored. Only three weeks before

Markingson committed suicide, Weiss had left an anguished voice message for the study coordinator, saying, "Do we have to wait until he kills himself or someone else before anyone does anything?"

The study in which Markingson died was funded by the pharmaceutical company AstraZeneca and designed to test its antipsychotic drug, Seroquel. The study was marked by alarming red flags: conflicts of interests, financial pressures to get subjects into the study, a locked psychiatric unit where severely ill patients were targeted for recruitment. Most disturbing of all were the conditions under which Markingson was enrolled. When he was admitted to Fairview, the university's teaching hospital, Markingson was in the grip of full-blown psychosis: delusional, confused, communicating with angels and aliens, convinced that he had been called to play a critical role in an apocalyptic mass murder event. Not only was Markingson psychotic when he signed the consent form, he was under a civil commitment order that legally required him to obey the recommendations of his psychiatrist. His mother wanted him to have nothing to do with the study. Olson enrolled Markingson anyway.

Some newspaper stories can be read with a measure of detachment, no matter how sad or horrifying they are. The characters are strangers, the setting a distant place. This story felt different. The study in which Markingson died took place at my own university. I had worked there for eleven years. I taught ethics in the medical school. I was friendly with faculty members in the Department of Psychiatry. For several years I had even been a member of the Institutional Review Board (IRB) that approved the study. Yet four years had passed since a suicidal research subject had tried to decapitate himself in a bathtub and I had heard nothing about it. How was that possible?

I knew that the Department of Psychiatry had a troubling

history. In the early 1990s, the head of child psychiatry had been sentenced to federal prison for research fraud.[2] Several years later, the Food and Drug Administration (FDA) had disqualified the director of the chemical dependency program for conducting an addiction experiment on illiterate Hmong opium addicts without their consent.[3] In 1997, the state medical board had suspended the license of a clinical faculty member after he was judged responsible for the injuries or deaths of forty-six mentally ill patients under his care, many of them in research studies.[4] But most of those incidents had occurred well before I arrived at the university.

The *Pioneer Press* series had included one small detail that especially bothered me. Mary Weiss had filed an unsuccessful lawsuit against the university. A judge ruled that because the University of Minnesota is a state institution, it had statutory immunity against this type of suit. Even if the university was at fault, it was protected against legal action. After winning that judgment, the university had struck back against Weiss with a "notice to assess costs," demanding that she pay the university over $56,000 to help settle its legal expenses.[5] That demand struck me as an act of petty cruelty. Reading that my own university had done this to a woman who had lost a son to suicide was the moment when I felt the first small flush of shame.

When I got back to Minnesota in August, I began to ask around about the *Pioneer Press* series. Almost no one had read it. Those who had didn't seem nearly as rattled by it as I was. The only people who seemed familiar with the controversy were either in the Department of Psychiatry or the university administration. Most of them were annoyed by my questions and bemused that I had taken a newspaper article seriously. More than once I was told that the *Pioneer Press* had treated the university unfairly and got the facts of the case wrong, although nobody could point to any specific fact that needed correction. It was suggested that if I wanted to blame anyone for the suicide, I should blame Mary Weiss.

Looking back on this period, I often wonder how the story might have played out if those conversations had gone differently. I simply assumed I would be taken seriously. It's not that I consider myself particularly formidable or believe that my personal convictions should be given special consideration. I just thought that the awful weight of the story, the sheer human tragedy of it, would give our conversations a measure of gravity. I wasn't prepared to be patronized. I didn't expect my comments to be met with eye-rolling and sighs. I didn't anticipate an introductory lecture on the necessity of the occasional human sacrifice on the long, glorious march of scientific progress. Would I have responded differently if someone had simply said something as meaningless as "Thank you for bringing these serious matters to our attention"? I can't say for certain. But if the purpose of those meetings was to intimidate me or deter me from looking further into the case, they had exactly the opposite effect.

Mary Weiss wasn't exactly eager to see anyone from the University of Minnesota, but after some assurances from Paul Tosto, she agreed to talk to me. We met in a coffee shop near Macalester College in St. Paul. Mary was an unimposing, white-haired woman with an Obama campaign pin on her jacket. Dan had been her only son. She had raised him as a single mother in St. Paul while working for the post office. Dan had been a gifted student, she told me. He had studied English literature at the University of Michigan and wanted to be a writer. When Dan had his first psychotic break in the summer of 2003, Mary had no idea what to do. She had no experience with mental illness. Her observations about the experience were measured and controlled, but her bitterness toward the university still seemed fresh.

In the conventional whistleblower narrative, an insider

asks, "Do I break with my group and speak out?" But the question facing me as I spoke to Mary was whether I should get involved in the first place. I wasn't really an insider. I had no more knowledge of this case than any other reader of the *Pioneer Press*. Like every other faculty member at the University of Minnesota, I had seen charges covered by the press without feeling any special obligation to insert myself into the controversy: financial corruption, sexual misconduct, an academic fraud scandal in the athletic department. Why should this case be any different?

That question has no simple answer. I felt terribly sorry for Mary Weiss; I felt ashamed of the way the university had treated her; I felt insulted by the way the administration had responded to me. I was also upset by the way the IRB had responded. It was hard to see how a committee charged with protecting the rights and welfare of human subjects could have looked seriously into Markingson's suicide without seeing the abuses the *Pioneer Press* identified. If our IRB had given an all clear to this study, how could anyone be certain that other research subjects had not been victimized as well?

If I am honest, I will admit that something about this case made it seem like a personal test. For years I had been highly critical of how comfortably the field of bioethics had embedded itself in the corridors of medical power. Bioethicists pretend they are watchdogs, I argued, but they act more like show dogs, groomed and displayed to assure the outside world that academic medicine takes ethics seriously. I had also leveled more than my share of criticism at the pharmaceutical industry, especially its perverse influence on medical research. The drug study in which Dan Markingson died was marked by the very abuses I had condemned. Could I really say nothing simply because those abuses took place at my own institution? I might as well put on a collar and beg for a treat.

To put it that way makes it sound as if speaking out was a

deliberate decision, like boarding a train to Canada. In reality I took a few halting steps in the dark that gradually led me over the border: a newspaper editorial, some class discussions, a brief appearance before the state legislature. There was one incident that now seems portentous. When I was invited to give a grand rounds lecture on ethics in the Department of Pediatrics, I included a short discussion of the Markingson case, hoping that other faculty members would find the facts of the case as upsetting as I did. But when the very first question was asked, I realized immediately how badly I had miscalculated. The audience was outraged, but not about the case. They were angry at me. The question-and-answer session felt like what sociologists call a "degradation ceremony," a public ritual designed to humiliate offenders and deviants. When it finally ended, I packed up my laptop and walked up the aisle toward the back of the lecture hall. No one would meet my eye. I remember fighting an intense desire to go back to my office, crawl under my desk, and open a bottle of Jack Daniels. It was 9 a.m.

In early 2009, a new finding emerged, this time from a different place. AstraZeneca was being sued for fraud by patients who had been prescribed Seroquel. Unsealed documents from that litigation showed that AstraZeneca had been manipulating research studies in order to make Seroquel look safer and more effective than it really was.[6] Company emails spoke of "cherry-picking" data and performing a "smoke-and-mirrors" job on it. Some of the manipulated studies apparently involved Charles Schulz, the chair of the University of Minnesota's Department of Psychiatry and a co-investigator on the study in which Dan Markingson died.[7]

As disturbing as the Markingson case was before, the possibility of research fraud made it even worse. What if Markingson had died in a study designed to be scientifically misleading? I approached an editor at the magazine *Mother*

Jones about the possibility of writing a story. When I got the go-ahead, I started digging as deeply as possible into the case, looking at medical records, depositions, expert testimony, unsealed memos, university records, anything I could find that seemed relevant. My naive hope was that national attention might shame the university into making amends or at least generate some public pressure for an external investigation.

Once again, I was wrong. When the article in *Mother Jones* appeared in the fall of 2010, it made virtually no public impact. The university didn't even respond until Minnesota Public Radio did a segment on the article, and when it did, the message was clear and dismissive. The university would not investigate further; there would be no more discussion; the case was closed. The only thing I had accomplished with the article was to alienate my employer and cement my growing reputation as a moralistic, self-righteous fanatic.

Looking back at this time, what strikes me is not just my naivete, which was considerable, but my complete misunderstanding of the situation. I knew that I wasn't winning any friends in the university administration. But I believed that tenure and the norms of academic freedom would insulate me from blowback. I assumed I could count on the support of my friends and colleagues in the Center for Bioethics. I thought my article in *Mother Jones* would find a sympathetic audience among the citizens of Minnesota, a state known for its progressive politics. About all of this I was badly mistaken. But my biggest mistake was to believe I was writing a story about research abuse rather than becoming a character in that story.

• • •

In novels and movies, the shape of the whistleblower narrative often resembles what Kurt Vonnegut called a "man-in-a-hole" story.[8] In these stories, someone gets into trouble and gets out again. Vonnegut used to plot the shape of the man-in-a-hole story on a graph: a straight line takes a deep dip and then returns to baseline. "People love that story," Vonnegut said. "They never get sick of it." The reason they love the story is because of its reassuring message. Job survives his ordeals and is rewarded by God for his faithfulness. Dorothy defeats the wicked witch and finds her way back to Kansas. The whistleblower exposes the truth and brings down the corrupt organization. The man gets out of the hole.

Missing are the lingering effects of being trapped in a hole. In the hole you turn inward. The world outside the hole fades away. Alone with your thoughts, you think of nothing but yourself and how to get out of the hole. The first time I met Mike Wilkins, the physician who blew the whistle on abusive conditions at the Willowbrook State School fifty years ago, we went out for breakfast at a diner in Minneapolis. Mike had struggled with mental health issues and wanted to hear about my experience. I gave him the man-in-a-hole version: what happened to Dan Markingson, what my friends and I did in response, how long and difficult our struggle was, and how we were eventually vindicated by two external investigations. But as I spoke, I could feel my voice harden and grow tense. I glanced down at my hands, which had tightened into clenched fists. When I finally finished, Mike just looked at me kindly and said, "You should probably get some therapy."

It has been over a decade since I tumbled headlong into the hole. Now that I've finally crawled out, it's painful to remember exactly what it was like at the bottom. Some days I woke up with a sense of gnawing anxiety, the sick feeling you get from a dream where you've been given a diagnosis of terminal cancer. It was never full-blown panic or fear, just the low background hum of dread. But I was also gripped by a kind of obsessiveness. No matter how hard I tried, I couldn't focus my attention on anything other than the Markingson case. Nothing was as important as what to do next: how to get the press involved, how to pry more information out of the university, how to mobilize public support, how to force the authorities to investigate. The sheer number of hours I wasted on efforts that would ultimately prove useless is staggering. I even understood this at the time, but still I couldn't stop, because nothing seemed to work and giving up was unthinkable.

The main barrier was the sheer intransigence of the university. It simply refused to engage with criticism on any level. Administrators would not discuss the case publicly other than to deny wrongdoing, and the university and hospital offices responsible for policing misconduct either stonewalled me or refused to investigate. Outside agencies were no better. The Office for Human Research Protection, the NIH, the FDA, the Minnesota attorney general's office, the Minnesota Board of Medical Practice, nonprofit organizations, civil liberties groups: no one was willing to help. I filed dozens of public records requests to the university, trying to learn if other research subjects had been mistreated. But the university had a seemingly limitless array of tactics to refuse or delay my requests: the document had been destroyed, the document was legally protected, the document could not be located, the document was available but only if I paid an exorbitant fee. These exchanges went on for years.

With each successive failure I sank deeper into the hole. Apparently, the only way to force the university's hand was to generate publicity about the case: petitions, letters, editorials, campus events, guest lectures, conference presentations, social media—anything to get attention. But attention was inevitably a mixed blessing. It shifted the controversy on campus from the case itself to my bizarre refusal to let it drop. Sometimes my newfound notoriety would get back to me secondhand: a dean who had blown up at the mention of my name, a friend who had diagnosed me as a "toxic narcissist," rumors that colleagues had been warned not to talk to me. More often the confrontations were direct. There were ominous threats, bitter arguments, formal complaints about my behavior filed to university authorities. People who had once been sympathetic began to turn away. The atmosphere in the Center for Bioethics grew so hostile that I felt uncomfortable going to my office. I began working mostly in coffee shops or at home, going into the university only to teach or meet with students.

I can remember a conversation from those years with Leigh Turner, a colleague in the Center for Bioethics and one of my closest friends. Leigh had moved to Minnesota from McGill University only a month or so after Markingson's death was exposed, and like me, he had watched the university's response with a growing sense of anger and disbelief. Leigh told me he felt like someone who had taken a job as a waiter only to discover that the restaurant was actually a front for a drug operation, like Los Pollos Hermanos in *Breaking Bad*. It hadn't taken long for Leigh to take up arms against the university—speaking out publicly, writing letters, filing lengthy complaints, confronting university officials. None of it worked. Soon Leigh was deep in the hole with me, trapped and desperate to find an exit. Without him, I'm not sure I would have survived.

In the spring of 2014, a few months before his eighty-second birthday, my father was hospitalized with a mysterious respiratory infection. A family doctor in solo practice for fifty-six years, he had still been seeing patients five days a week when he got sick. After a couple of weeks in the hospital, he finally improved enough to be moved to an acute rehabilitation unit. I flew home to South Carolina to help. One morning I noticed that he was nodding off during breakfast. A nurse checked his vitals and discovered that his blood pressure was dangerously low. Immediately he was rushed to the ICU and placed on a sepsis protocol: a ventilator, vasopressors, fluids, and IV antibiotics. Blood cultures later revealed that he had Legionnaires' disease, a rare bacterial infection that is usually spread through aerosolized water systems, such as air-conditioning units.

For the next six months, my father lurched from one near-lethal episode to another: sepsis, pneumonias, viral ulcers, unexpected drug side effects, urinary tract infections, long stretches on a ventilator, a tracheostomy, a gastrostomy tube, an infected pain pump, and a critical care specialist who insisted repeatedly that we should just allow him to die. This period was so dark that I still can't talk about it without a sense of physical queasiness. It was as if our entire family had been strapped into a roller coaster that was careening out of control. The ordeal would have probably killed most eighty-two-year-olds, but my father had a deep reservoir of resilience, an unwavering faith in medical science, and a bizarrely high tolerance for pain. Twice he survived life-threatening episodes of septic shock, and each time he left the ICU we shook our heads in astonishment. This must be how Martha felt when Lazarus emerged from the tomb. Yet still we lived every day on a knife's edge, because we never knew how long the resurrection would last.

None of us were mentally prepared for this ordeal. My father had always been the person my brothers and I looked to reflexively in a crisis, simply because he was such a competent human being. Now he was utterly dependent and vulnerable. Our mother fell apart. Her attitude swung wildly between cheerfully inappropriate denial and crushing emotional devastation. My own state of mind was a mix of despair, anxiety, and boiling rage at anyone I saw as an enemy—the university bureaucrats who were tormenting me, the former friends and colleagues in the Center for Bioethics who had turned against me, the smirking doctor at the nursing home whose indifference sent my father back to the hospital in septic shock. My memory of that period is a haze of sickening dread, panicked last-second flights to South Carolina, and ugly confrontations with doctors and administrators, all of it compounded by a growing fear that even if my father survived, he would never be the same. Just as I thought that the situation at the university could not possibly get worse, I found myself sleeping in a recliner in the ICU.

When you are deep in the hole, the darkness makes it hard to know who to trust. The more notoriety the Markingson case achieved, the more I was sought out by strangers: psychiatric survivors, patient advocates, would-be whistleblowers, civil libertarians, anti-pharma activists, Scientologists, and conspiracy theorists of every possible variety. Some people wanted to thank me. Others came with confidential advice or secret information. Many were seeking help. Their communications came in every imaginable form: phone calls, voice messages, handwritten notes, emails, social media, anonymous letters, self-published books, mysterious packages, lengthy personal accounts of abuse at the hands of psychiatrists. One poor man who turned up at my office was so paranoid that he was afraid to tell me his name. Several were faculty members with their own alarming accounts of mistreatment by university officials.

One message came from a former patient at Fairview Hospital named Robert Huber. When we spoke on the phone, he told me a story of psychiatric mistreatment that sounded disturbingly similar to that of Dan Markingson. After going to the emergency room with symptoms of psychosis, Huber had been involuntarily confined to a locked psychiatric unit. Like Markingson, he was seen by Stephen Olson, who proceeded to recruit him into a drug study. The study was funded by a pharmaceutical company and designed to test an experimental antipsychotic drug called bifeprunox. Huber said that he was told that unless he signed up for the study, he would face very large medical bills. He had never taken an antipsychotic drug before, much less an experimental one. Like Markingson, Huber became suicidal. Unlike Markingson, he managed to drop out of the study without killing himself.

I put Robert Huber in touch with Jeff Baillon, an investigative reporter for KMSP television who had begun looking into the university's Department of Psychiatry and Behavioral Sciences. In May 2014, after hospital records confirmed Huber's story, KMSP ran a detailed segment on the case.[9] Huber and I each filed formal complaints. But the university didn't budge. Several months later a hospital whistleblower stepped forward. Niki Gjere, a senior psychiatric nurse and patient safety specialist, told KMSP that nurses at Fairview had been badgered into enrolling patients into psychiatric studies.[10] Back in 2003 she had objected to enrolling Markingson in the Astra-Zeneca study, arguing that he was too vulnerable, but her objections had been ignored. Speaking to a television reporter did not make Niki a popular figure at Fairview. Soon she joined Leigh and me in the hole.

The occupational hazard of whistleblowing is an inability to stop ruminating over the past, mentally rehearsing every battle and betrayal in order to convince yourself that you acted honorably. I still feel that impulse, but I don't really have the stomach for it anymore. It's not that I regret taking up the cause. I still feel that Dan Markingson should be alive. I still believe that my university treated Mary Weiss with terrible cruelty. But I'm not proud of the person I became during that time. The struggle twisted me in ways that I would not have imagined. Just the thought of it makes me uncomfortable: my paranoia and self-pity; my dark, volatile moods at home; the misplaced trust I placed in people I mistakenly saw as allies; my dismissive attitude toward colleagues I viewed as hopelessly naive; all the futile gestures that I made in the desperate hope that they might advance the cause, but which now seem ridiculous and embarrassing. Did I actually build a black coffin for a group of students in white coats to carry into a meeting of the Board of Regents? Did I really imagine it would help the cause to tweet out a photograph of my twelve-year-old daughter, Lyle, holding a guinea pig while wearing a rubber pig mask and a University of Minnesota lab coat with money spilling out of the pockets?

I know what you're thinking. Anybody who claims he isn't confrontational but spends seven years picking ridiculous fights in public is either lying or deluded. To be honest, I find it hard to explain. All I can tell you is that I was gripped by an obsession that would not turn loose. I come from a long line of hardheaded Presbyterian women and stubborn Southern men. By writing the *Mother Jones* article and refusing to let the issue drop, I had turned myself into a public figure whose entire reputation seemed to rest on a single issue. If I surrendered, I would be seen not just as a vindictive traitor, but as a vindictive traitor who was wrong. Giving up without any success whatsoever would have meant that everything I had done up to that point had amounted to nothing more than pushing the self-destruct button. That was an outcome I was unable to consider.

· · ·

If you are writing a man-in-a-hole story, you know from the start that the man will get out of the hole. Getting him out of the hole is the entire point of the story. You know exactly how the graph will look, when the line will dip and when it will rise again. But when you're a character in that story, you have no idea what kind of story you're in, much less how it ends. You don't know if you're in a hole, or a tunnel, or a crawl space underneath a serial killer's porch steps. All you know is that you're flailing around in the dark. Even if you finally make your way out of the hole, it may not be obvious until much later how it happened. Did you escape or were you rescued?

In April 2013, I came across a scathing editorial in the *Star Tribune* by Arne Carlson, a former Republican governor of Minnesota whose second term had ended in 1998.[11] Carlson was upset with the excessive salaries that senior administrators at the University of Minnesota were paying themselves. Although I didn't know much about Carlson, I could see that he was angry with the very same people I had been fighting against for years. So I sent him a note by email, along with some material about the Markingson case. I didn't imagine he would reply; I had sent the very same note to a state legislator and to the director of a local mental health nonprofit, both of whom had ignored it. To my astonishment, Arne Carlson replied right away. Should we talk about this over breakfast? Absolutely, I said. Just tell me where to go. Carlson replied: Meet me at Perkins in Golden Valley.

When the appointed time arrived, I packed up a folder of documents and drove to a chain restaurant in the suburbs for hash browns and scrambled eggs with the ex-governor. I spotted him sitting alone in a booth, hunched over the table like Humphrey Bogart. Our meeting started with the feeling of a deposition. Governor Carlson had a number of pointed questions for me. He took notes and listened carefully. He made it clear that he had a zero tolerance policy for evasiveness, pretension, or bullshit. This suited me fine, since I have a very similar policy. After fifteen minutes or so, his manner began to soften. He dropped his guard and told a few stories, some of them at his own expense. He was opinionated, sardonic, and very funny. I decided I liked him. But I couldn't tell whether I had won his trust.

After our second pot of coffee, my kidneys kicked into gear. When I excused myself to go to the bathroom, I heard a voice from a nearby booth: "Carl!" It was Paul Quie, a retired physician I knew from the university. A kind, old-school pediatrician, Paul had been instrumental in setting up the Center for

Bioethics decades earlier. He asked what I was doing at Perkins. "Believe it or not, I'm having breakfast with the ex-governor," I said. "Well, so am I," Paul told me. "Do you know my brother, Al?" Sitting across the table was Al Quie, a Republican governor of Minnesota from the early 1980s. Within minutes Arne and Al were clapping each other on the back and talking about the old days.

If Kurt Vonnegut were plotting this story on a graph, he would mark "Perkins in Golden Valley" as a point where the line started curving upward. Arne and I left the restaurant as friends. For the next two years, he threw himself into the cause with the force of a middle linebacker. He wrote editorials. He called legislators. He gave interviews to the press. He met with Eric Kaler, the university president. The more resistance Arne encountered, the more determined he became. The fight seemed to energize him. As governor, Arne had been a tremendous supporter of the university. He had even worn a University of Minnesota letter jacket for his official portrait. That record of support gave special force to his blistering attacks on Kaler, who had asked to meet with Arne but refused to meet privately with me or Leigh. Almost as important as Arne's public support was his private encouragement. He was relentlessly upbeat. He often called me several times a week to plot strategy, to share news, to insist that we would eventually prevail. It was like having a fantastically confident basketball coach.

For a long time, I couldn't see any change. If anything, the university seemed even more unyielding than before. Dan Markingson had died in 2004. By the time Arne and I had breakfast at Perkins nine years later, most of the key administrative positions at the university were held by people with no involvement at all in the original case. It seemed reasonable to think that they might look at the controversy with a degree of objectivity. Yet every person who stepped into a new adminis-

trative position behaved just as their predecessors had. It was
as if each one had been left a detailed manual instructing them
how to avoid dealing with the case.

One administrative position that hadn't changed for two
decades was that of the general counsel. Beginning in the early
1990s, Mark Rotenberg had steered the university through a
seemingly endless series of lawsuits, controversies, and public
scandals, including the Markingson case. But in June of 2013,
Rotenberg told the university that he was leaving Minnesota
for a position at Johns Hopkins University. When the university announced a celebration in his honor, I decided to go.
Why exactly, I can't say. Perhaps I entertained secret thoughts
of interrupting the feast, like Banquo's ghost. More likely it
was just morbid curiosity. Although I regarded Rotenberg as a
mortal enemy, I had never seen him in person.

When the time for celebration arrived, I lurked silently on
the sidelines, watching as one speaker after another ascended
the platform to praise Rotenberg's legal brilliance and moral
integrity. My blood pressure climbed upward. I cursed under
my breath. I fantasized about rushing the stage. After an hour
or so standing up, I decided to rest on the ledge of a shallow
reflecting pool that ran along one wall. What I thought was
a ledge, however, was actually part of the pool. I sat down in
water about 2 inches deep. Slowly I got back to my feet, the
back of my pants dripping wet, and looked around to see if anyone had witnessed my humiliation. Then I carefully backed
out of the room.

It wasn't easy to summon up hope. Yet as the months
passed, a few faint flickers of light began to appear in the darkness. By the fall of 2014, two separate investigations of the university were underway. One was the work of Arne Carlson. As
a liberal Republican who often endorsed Democrats for public office, Arne could exert political leverage in unexpected
places, one of which was the higher education committee of

the state senate. Somehow Arne had convinced the committee to ask the Office of the Legislative Auditor to investigate the Markingson case. The Office of the Legislative Auditor is a nonpartisan watchdog agency that serves the legislature. It is probably the most respected government bureau in the state. There was reason to believe it would conduct a fair investigation.

The second investigation was taking place on campus. The initiative for that investigation had come from Trudo Lemmens, an old friend who held a chair in health law at the University of Toronto. Trudo had recruited 170 experts in health law and bioethics to ask the University of Minnesota's Faculty Senate to investigate Markingson's death. Armed with Trudo's letter, a group of campus allies who served as senators from the College of Liberal Arts had pushed through a formal resolution calling for such an investigation. President Kaler had refused to comply, but as a concession to public pressure, he had agreed to an external review of the university's research oversight program. It would be conducted by the Association for the Accreditation of Human Research Protection Programs.

By Thanksgiving, my father had finally recovered enough to move back home with my mother. For over six months he had been shifted back and forth between a hospital, a long-term acute care facility, an acute rehabilitation unit, and a nursing home. Although he still needed a wheelchair and a gastrostomy tube, the immediate danger to his health had passed and his cognition was back to normal. It felt like a small miracle. We arranged a hospital bed, a disability ramp, a motorized wheelchair, and home health care. With some assistance, it looked as if he and my mother could manage on their own again. My brothers and I could stop holding our breaths.

If this were a man-in-a-hole story, this would be the point at which I describe how I finally emerged from the hole, coughing and squinting in the sunlight. It began in the early months of 2015. On February 27, the university reluctantly released the external review it had commissioned.[12] While the language of the report was careful, the content was damning. Not only did the report find major flaws and weaknesses in the university's research oversight program, but it also identified an alarming "culture of fear" in the Department of Psychiatry, where staff members were frightened of retaliation if they brought up concerns about patient safety.[13]

Three weeks later, the Office of the Legislative Auditor (OLA) delivered what *MinnPost* called a "stunning rebuke" to the university.[14] The OLA report read like an indictment. Released in a public session at the state capitol, it blasted the university for the way it had handled the Markingson case, citing coercive recruitment practices, financial conflicts of interest, and superficial ethical reviews. It also singled out university leaders for their misleading public statements and their refusal to acknowledge criticism or ethical scrutiny.[15] President Kaler was finally forced to answer for the university's intransigence in public.

But I'm not sure this is a man-in-a-hole story. What I had failed to understand was that public vindication is not the same as getting out of the hole. It's more like crawling out of a ditch in the middle of a desert. After those two critical reports were released, nothing much changed at the university. No one was fired or punished. Nobody admitted personal fault. There was no genuine apology to Mary Weiss, who suffered a stroke in 2011 and had become increasingly frail, just a grudging statement that did not admit fault.[16]

Financial compensation was never even discussed. Robert Huber was forgotten; the university never admitted any serious misconduct in his case. Leigh and I remained just as isolated on campus as we had always been. There were no apologies, no mea culpas, no admissions that we had done the

right thing. No physician at the university expressed sympathy or solidarity, even in private. If anything, public vindication simply made most people in the academic health center
despise us even more.

Does that assessment sound bitter? I don't mean to suggest that nothing was accomplished. The university administration agreed to a temporary suspension of psychiatric drug
studies. It set up a research reform task force. A few weeks
after the *New York Times* reported yet another ethically ques-
tionable drug study in the Department of Psychiatry, Charles
Schulz announced that he would be retiring as chair of the
department (while continuing to remain employed as a senior
faculty member).[17] Yet none of these things felt like what we
had hoped for. They seemed more like public relations tactics
devised to mollify the state legislature. A year after the external reports were released, a review of the Department of Psychiatry found that little had changed for the better.[18]

When Kurt Vonnegut plotted out the shapes of stories, not
all the shapes ended with an upward curve. Some stories went
from bad to worse. If you're working at a pedestrian job and
wake up one morning to find yourself transformed into a giant
beetle, the line on the graph starts at a low point and plum-
mets dramatically. Many Old Testament stories have a similar
trajectory. The line starts at zero, and maybe it curves slightly
upward for a while. But eventually there comes a spectacular
fall: Lot's wife is turned into salt, Adam and Eve are expelled
from Eden, Jezebel is thrown out of the window and eaten by
dogs. It's different in the New Testament, where most stories
end with an upward curve. But there is at least one notable
exception, and it doesn't end well for the whistleblower.

• • •

When spring comes to South Carolina, the Judas trees are
hard to miss. It's not that they are especially large or beauti-

fully shaped. I've seen far more Judas trees growing wild on the side of the road than I have seen in anyone's yard. But their scraggly branches are covered in flaming purple-pink flowers, and sometimes they jut out at odd angles, like a crayon picture of a man whose hair is on fire. Judas trees often bloom around Easter, but exactly why they're named for Judas—rather than, say, Peter or John or even Jesus himself—I've never quite understood. As children, we were told that Judas Iscariot hanged himself from one of those trees after he betrayed Jesus, but that explanation never made much sense, not unless the Judas trees are a lot sturdier in Jerusalem. Most of our Judas trees are more like big Judas bushes. You can't really hang anything on them much heavier than a bird feeder.

The story of Judas looms over any act of disloyalty. Peter may have denied Jesus, and Thomas may have doubted him, but Judas was the disciple who betrayed him with a kiss. Even worse, he did it for cash, selling Jesus out for thirty pieces of silver. The Gospel of Matthew says that later, when Jesus was condemned to death, Judas was so consumed by guilt for his betrayal that he gave the money back and hanged himself. In *The Divine Comedy*, Judas is the most tormented person in hell. When Virgil gives Dante his tour of the inner circle, they see Lucifer frozen in ice, the torso of Judas dangling out of one of his three mouths. It seems safe to conclude that early Christians didn't look kindly on institutional insiders who turned against the organization.

Nor do most academic physicians. Doctors like to think of themselves as hard-nosed empiricists, but the culture of academic medicine is as closed and insular as the medieval church. It is rigidly hierarchical. It is governed by ritual and ceremony. It commands deep respect from the community, yet it has secrets that the community can't be permitted to know. Like the church, academic medicine has a moral mission that is protected by a complex set of orthodoxies and articles of faith. At the heart of this moral mission is medical research, the practice that is rewarded above all others. Research is what funds the enterprise, what launches faculty members up the hierarchy, and what distinguishes academic physicians from lesser doctors practicing in the community. To question the value of medical research is heresy. To expose its abuses is an act of treachery so grave that it will propel you headfirst into the mouth of Lucifer.

Not that anyone really needs Dante to instruct them on the morality of betrayal. Most of us learn it as soon as we can speak. The English words used to characterize people who turn against the group are almost uniformly disparaging. We call them traitors, backstabbers, turncoats, treasonists, and Benedict Arnolds. To describe people who disclose unwelcome information about the group, we deploy a larger and more specialized vocabulary: snitches, squealers, narcs, rats, tattletales, finks, and stool pigeons. Against this chorus of moral condemnation, only the relatively recent neologism "whistleblower" conveys any sense that turning on your own group might be an admirable course of action. But well intentioned though "whistleblower" may be, it transmits none of the visceral moral power of a word like "rat" or "snitch." The image evoked by "whistleblower" is likely to be a puffing referee in a striped uniform or maybe a lowly traffic cop waving his hands at an intersection.

Like anyone else who has engaged in a morally controversial act, whistleblowers need a story to tell themselves about their experience. Ending that story with an upward curve can be a struggle. Things do not usually go well for whistleblowers themselves, and their actions rarely generate lasting institutional change. Whistleblowers in search of a hopeful ending must often find a way of putting a morally positive spin on an act of betrayal whose consequences have been outwardly disastrous. They need to tell a story of heroic sacrifice in ser-

vice of a just cause, or of a righteous struggle against an unfor-
giving world, or the higher rewards of remaining true to your
principles. Otherwise, their story risks looking like that of
Judas as told in the Gospel of Matthew.

In the novel *My Name was Judas,* the New Zealand writer
C. K. Stead imagines a story of betrayal told by Judas himself.[19]
In Stead's version, Judas didn't hang himself or take any silver.
Nor did he betray Jesus with a kiss. Like the other disciples,
Judas left Jerusalem when Jesus was executed, eventually set-
tling in a Greek community in Sidon. There he raised a family
and lived happily under the name Idas of Sidon. Forty years
later, Judas is looking back on his friendship with Jesus. He
explains how the cult of personality surrounding Jesus arose
and how things spiraled so badly out of control.

This Judas was no ordinary disciple. He and Jesus had
been close childhood friends, tutored by the same teacher.
Judas came from privilege, the grandson of a rabbi and the
son of a prosperous trader, while Jesus was a clever, charming boy from humble origins who grew into a charismatic religious leader and social activist. Jesus spoke like a poet and
a prophet, championing the poor and the oppressed. When
Judas lost his wife and unborn child, Jesus invited him to join
his group on the road as they traveled and advocated for social
change. Grief-stricken and lost, Judas said yes.

But Judas never really fit in. Some of the disciples were
uneducated fishermen. Others just seemed deranged. Judas
found himself uncomfortable with the air of worshipfulness
surrounding Jesus. The disciples sounded like a bickering
royal court, vying for the favors of the prince, and they had
an unnerving habit of exaggeration. If a crowd shared their
meals, stretching their portions so that everyone could eat, it
wasn't just a testament to human goodness; it was a miracle
performed by Jesus, who had fed the five thousand with fishes
and loaves. If Jesus persuaded an emaciated, dispirited man to

get out of his bed, it was not just ministering to the sick; it was a miracle in which Jesus had brought a dead man back to life. Even more disturbing was the way Jesus tolerated the exaggerations with a gentle smile. He didn't even correct the disciples when they called him the Messiah.

According to Judas, there was never a single episode of betrayal. Over time, the compassionate Jesus, champion of the oppressed, transformed himself into Jesus the revolutionary, a fiery militant who chased the money changers out of the Temple and called out the Pharisees as parasites and hypocrites. Judas worried constantly about this transformation. Jesus seemed unaware of how politically dangerous his activism had become. At times his sermons were so grandiose that Judas thought Jesus was veering into mental illness. Judas tried to warn him, but Jesus was in no position to hear advice anymore. While Judas never opposed Jesus directly, the mere tone of his comments pushed the two men apart. Judas says, "My silences were enough to tell him where I stood, and also to make it clear to the other disciples, who were constantly demanding to know why I would not affirm this or that about the Master's powers and his greatness."[20]

So that was the betrayal: not a kiss, not a bag of silver, just a quiet reluctance to conform to the demands of the group. When it all ended as badly as Judas had feared, he left Jerusalem in disgust, not just with the gruesome execution but with his failure to save Jesus from himself. Over the decades he has looked on from Sidon as the myths about Jesus grew, especially those told about his own role in the story. "At the end of their narration I always die—sometimes by my own hand (a barren fig tree seems to be a favoured site), or in a horrible accident in which I fall down in a field with the money the betrayal of Jesus earned me," Judas says. "In this version I'm split open on a ploughshare and my blood and intestines spill out over the ground, which at once becomes infertile."[21]

As the public controversy over the Markingson case died away, I struggled to tell myself a coherent story about what had happened. Part of the problem was the absence of any clear resolution. Not a bang, not a whimper, just the pretense of a truce. How do you prosecute a campaign against an enemy who has pretended to lay down his arms? For years I had been telling a story about the mistreatment of Dan Markingson to others in hopes of forcing a legitimate investigation. Now that the investigations had come and gone, I had to reckon with the part I had played. I didn't feel like Judas as he is portrayed in the Bible. I have never felt the deep loyalty of medicine's true believers, and I wasn't tortured with guilt over betraying my organization. I felt more like the Judas in Stead's novel, uncomfortable around zealots, reflexively suspicious when the group is too certain of its own righteousness, even when the group is my own.

Yet I am self-aware enough to understand my own tendency toward smug self-righteousness. I may not be confrontational, but I have a contrarian streak, an impatience with accepted truths that sometimes leads me to places that I regret. And while I had no doubt that the University of Minnesota had behaved disgracefully, I winced every time I thought back about myself as the public face of the opposition, lecturing and hectoring the wicked like Jonathan Edwards in the pulpit. What gnawed at me was not just anxiety about my moral arrogance but a feeling of self-recrimination about my mistakes. Surely it could all have gone better. Maybe if I had taken the time to study whistleblowing more carefully before I launched myself into a moral crusade, I wouldn't feel so demoralized and ambivalent about the result.

In order to educate myself, I began teaching an honors seminar for undergraduates on medical research scandals. I've taught the seminar for over seven years now, updating the syllabus as new research scandals come to light. We typically start by looking at the notorious scandals exposed in the 1960s and '70s and then continue through to present-day cases. Exploitation of the homeless, the imprisoned, the poor, and the uneducated; studies of schizophrenia, cervical cancer, leukemia, syphilis, hepatitis, and starvation; death by suicide, sepsis, and surgical misadventure. The class is a brutal, nonstop highlight reel of deception and abuse. My aim in teaching it is to examine these research scandals side by side to see if there are any common elements. How do they usually play out?

The short answer is: very badly. Research institutions do not readily admit fault, even when it is glaringly obvious, and rarely do mistreated research subjects or their families get any real justice. Whistleblowing is the exception, not the rule. In many scandals, doctors and other staff members remained silent for years while unwitting research subjects were abused. In many cases, the dissenters who dared to blow the whistle disappeared from public sight a long time ago. These people often seem like ghosts haunting the memory of the studies, vanished and forgotten. Why had they chosen to act when so many others did nothing? What kind of stories had they told themselves to make sense of their ordeal?

This book is a conversation with the ghosts. I began writing it in an effort to climb out of the hole, thinking that maybe I could wrench my attention away from my own troubles by turning it toward those of others. I have tried to do their stories justice, but that was not my only aim. I also wanted to use those stories as a vehicle for exploring larger questions that I wish I had understood better before I embarked on my own crusade. It was my hope that by looking at these stories alongside each other, I could see patterns emerge that might help others undergoing similar struggles.

Whether I have succeeded is for others to judge. I would have liked to conclude the book with an inspirational message, perhaps one that would encourage potential whistleblowers to speak out. But ending the book that way would have felt dishonest. If there are lessons in these whistleblower stories, they are much more ambiguous and provisional. The threads that run through them will become evident as I tell them: the power of social conformity, the importance of solidarity, the necessity of perseverance, and the lingering sense of disillusionment that many whistleblowers can't seem to shake. What struck me most of all were the extraordinary efforts to which these whistleblowers went to hold onto their souls, to emerge from the hole with a sense of honor and personal integrity.

As I spoke with the whistleblowers, I sometimes found myself wondering how their stories would compare with those of the people who stood by and did nothing as the abuses unfolded. What kinds of stories would these bystanders tell? Maybe, like the gospel writers, they would tell a story in which they remained faithful to a moral cause while the whistleblower betrayed them out of greed or resentment. Perhaps they would portray themselves as hard-nosed scientists capable of moving beyond weepy sentimentalism for the sake of the greater good. Or maybe they would have simply forgotten about the abuses. Most of us have a remarkable ability to avoid thinking about unpleasant events, especially ones in which we have behaved in unflattering ways. It is possible that bad behavior had become so routine and ordinary that it simply blended into the wallpaper. Over time everyone stopped seeing the stain.

Yet what sets these whistleblowers apart from bystanders is not simply that they saw moral wrongs for what they were. It is that speaking out about the abuses was a real possibility for them, an action it occurred to them to take. For many people, blowing the whistle is a thought that never enters the mind. When I look back at myself in medical school, what separates me from the person I was back then isn't really a difference in moral perception. Even then I knew, deep down, that it was wrong to perform a pelvic exam on a non-consenting unconscious woman or to attempt an invasive procedure that I was unqualified to perform simply because I was told to do it. What didn't occur to me back then was the possibility of resistance.

Like Judas in C. K. Stead's novel, I am still trying to tell a meaningful story about my experience. That has meant thinking about alternative stories: what I feel proud of and what I regret, the different choices I might have made, how my life might have gone if I had decided not to get involved. It has helped to talk to others who have gone through similar ordeals. Some of us are looking for the sermon in the suicide, as Joan Didion famously put it, while others have no patience for such philosophical nonsense. Everyone has a different story to tell. I would like mine to end on an upward curve.

The Honor Code

For Christmas a few years ago, my daughter Martha made a sign for the door of my office. It features a silhouette of our thirty-seventh president and bears the heading "Institute for Nixon Studies." Like the rest of my family, Martha thinks I'm obsessed with Richard Nixon. In my office are 1972 campaign posters, bookshelves lined with Watergate books, LP records of speeches by Nixon and Spiro Agnew, and a rubber Nixon mask sitting on the neck of my bass guitar. Maybe it looks obsessive, but I say take your inspiration where you find it. Personally, I never thought an Enemies List was such a bad idea.

Nixon is not so much an obsession as a permanent fixture of my psychological architecture. In May of 1973, when the Senate Watergate Committee began its hearings, I was eleven years old. For hours on end there was nothing else on television. It is tempting to call Watergate my first real political memory, but the word "memory" doesn't really do justice to its ontological status. The whole episode feels more like a

weird dream. The villains were mythic: the sneering Ehrlichman, the stone-faced Mitchell, the supersquare Bob Haldeman with his military brush cut, and of course the Dark One
himself, sweating in the Oval Office and cursing the hippies.
By the time Nixon resigned in 1974, the drama had burrowed
its way deep into my unconscious and settled somewhere next
to *The Wizard of Oz* and the more disturbing parts of the King
James Bible.

Watergate was the ultimate whistleblowing story in an era
packed full of them. In 1968, Ernest Fitzgerald, of the Pentagon, testified to a Senate subcommittee about a $2.3 billion
cost overrun. In 1969, Ron Ridenhour wrote to Nixon and
members of Congress about the massacre of innocent Viet-
namese civilians by his fellow American soldiers at My Lai.
In 1970, Frank Serpico gave the *New York Times* secret information about corruption in the New York City police department. In 1971, Daniel Ellsberg leaked the Pentagon Papers. All
these men spoke out for morally admirable reasons and suffered for it.

Yet nothing of that period has ever quite reached the status of the Watergate scandal and the figures who exposed it:
Alexander Butterfield, the Nixon aide who told the Senate
about the secret White House taping system; John Dean, the
White House attorney who turned state's witness and testified
against his bosses; and of course, Mark Felt, aka Deep Throat,
the shadowy figure who guided Bob Woodward and Carl Bernstein through their investigations for the *Washington Post* and
whose identity remained secret for thirty years. Each acted for
different reasons and used different methods; each suffered a
different fate. None of them were whistleblowers in the strict
sense of the word, but their actions helped clarify what the
concept of whistleblower would come to mean.

It is unlikely that any of the Watergate-era figures we now
call whistleblowers would have even used that term. Until the

early 1970s, the term *whistleblower* was virtually unknown. For Taylor Branch and Charles Peters, who published one of the first major books on whistleblowing in 1972, the term represented a conscious effort to redescribe people who had previously been called "traitors" or "rats." Branch and Peters called the whistleblower a "muckraker from within, who exposes what he considers the unconscionable practices of his own organization."[1] They didn't distinguish between insiders who blow the whistle to save their own necks and those whose motives were selfless. Nor did they distinguish between whistleblowers who had gone public and those who had leaked damaging information in secret. Their main distinction was between "pure" whistleblowers, who expose wrongdoing in an organization where they are working, and "alumni" whistleblowers, who blow the whistle after they leave.

For decades the most celebrated figure involved in exposing Watergate was Deep Throat, the anonymous source eventually identified as the associate director of the FBI, Mark Felt. In their 1974 book, *All the President's Men,* Woodward and Bernstein portrayed Deep Throat as a straight-arrow Washington insider exhausted by endless political fights.[2] Deep Throat was deeply concerned about the cutthroat tactics of the Nixon White House. "They are all underhanded and unknowable," he told Woodward, calling their eagerness to fight dirty a "switchblade mentality." Paranoid about secrecy, Deep Throat communicated with Woodward using cloak-and-dagger techniques that could have been lifted from John le Carré. When Woodward needed to meet Deep Throat, he moved a flowerpot with a red flag to the rear of his apartment balcony. When Deep Throat needed to meet Woodward, a hand-drawn clock with the appointed time would appear on page 20 of Woodward's copy of the *New York Times.* The two men met late at night in an underground parking garage.

Deep Throat didn't blow the whistle, of course. He took the

quiet, time-honored route favored by Washington insiders: the strategic leak. Because leakers do not identify themselves publicly, leaking has a more morally fraught status than whistleblowing. Some leakers act for honorable reasons; Daniel Ellsberg leaked the Pentagon Papers to the press because he had learned that the American government was lying to the public about the war in Vietnam. (Later he outed himself and became a full-fledged whistleblower.) But other leakers act for reasons that are self-serving. In fact, many leaks—or rather, "leaks"—are sanctioned by an organization and intended merely to manipulate the press. Maybe Felt was motivated by righteous outrage at Nixon's corruption, but if he had leaked for selfish reasons, such as to damage an enemy, he wouldn't have been the first agent in J. Edgar Hoover's FBI to do it. As Max Holland has written, "No federal agency rivaled the FBI in terms of the well-placed, exquisitely timed disclosure designed with an end in mind."[3]

In May 1973, nobody outside the *Washington Post* had heard of Deep Throat. Yet everyone watching the Watergate hearings had an opinion about John Dean, Nixon's inscrutable White House counsel and a key player in the scandal. Dean's horn-rimmed glasses gave him the look of an accountant, but he spoke like a cold-blooded assassin. He spilled everything: the bugging of Democratic National Committee headquarters, the cover-up, the payoff to Howard Hunt, the infamous Enemies List. It wasn't clear if he could be believed. Unlike many of the other figures in Watergate, Dean was virtually unknown to the public before the Watergate hearings. Hunter Thompson, an admirer, called him a "fiendish drone." He wrote, "Dean radiates a certain, very narrow kind of authority—nothing personal, but the kind of nasal blank-hearted authority you feel in the presence of the taxman or a very polite FBI agent."[4]

Dean was telling the truth, of course, and for that he has

been rightly celebrated. But in 1973, most people saw him as a traitor, including many liberals. Writing in the *New York Review of Books*, Nicholas von Hoffman said that Dean was "the American ratfink of the twentieth century, so much so that a century hence 'to pull a John Dean' may mean to double-cross your pals."[5] The press portrayed him as a sleazy political operative who had weaseled his way upward in the White House by sucking up to his bosses only to squeal in hopes of avoiding a prison sentence. Joseph Alsop famously called him a "bottom-dwelling slug." Dean himself understood why; he was complicit in the crimes he was exposing. "No one likes a squealer, a Judas, an informant, a tattletale, especially one who is also guilty," he wrote in his memoir.[6]

Loyalty is a Boy Scout virtue, and nobody feels the pain of disloyalty more acutely than whistleblowers themselves. Of all the crimes and sins that Dean committed in the White House—destroying evidence, punishing political enemies, obstructing justice—it was the prospect of disloyalty that seared his conscience most. Dean had worked under Attorney General John Mitchell and felt very close to him. Not only had Mitchell approved the Watergate break-in, but he had also admitted it to Dean. For Dean to tell the truth about Watergate would mean a prison sentence for Mitchell, a man he thought of as an uncle. "Now I felt the razor edge between the squealer and the perjurer," Dean wrote. "I had never felt more squalid."[7]

Perhaps the most honorable figure to emerge from Watergate was Alexander Butterfield, one of the few staffers who knew about Nixon's secret taping system in the Oval Office. Unlike Dean, Butterfield was involved in no illegal activity. Unlike Felt, he had no career ambitions that would be served by his revelations. Butterfield simply found it impossible to lie. When he was asked a direct question about Nixon's tapes during the Watergate hearings, he answered honestly. "Are you aware of the installation of any listening devices in the Oval Office?" Fred Thompson, the minority counsel for the Senate Watergate Committee, asked Butterfield. "I was aware of listening devices, yes, sir," Butterfield said, after a pause. With that single sentence, Butterfield handed over the keys to the Watergate cover-up.

Butterfield never wanted to betray Nixon. In later interviews, he explained that if he had not been asked about the secret taping system, he would not have volunteered the information. Nor did he face the prospect of betrayal without fear. He knew that all three television networks were broadcasting the hearings live. "I was pretty aware that moment could change my life. I thought I could be drummed out of the Nixon administration immediately," Butterfield said. "I'm thinking how much time do I have to pack a bag and leave town." He remembered going into the restroom before the hearings, washing his face, and pausing in front of the mirror for a second or two. Butterfield didn't know exactly what he was going to say. "But I knew I was going to answer questions and I knew I wasn't going to have any trouble answering them."[8]

Whistleblowers are often asked why they spoke up despite the grave risks to themselves. Their answers are often disarmingly matter-of-fact. They don't make complex moral arguments. They don't appeal to foundational principles. They don't cite legal statutes or verses from the Bible. They say things like "I had to be able to look at myself in the mirror" or "That's simply how I was raised." When Butterfield was asked why he answered honestly, he said that the decision wasn't really conscious. "I answered truthfully because I am a truthful person," Butterfield explained. "I simply knew I wouldn't lie. I would never lie," he said. "This may sound a little corny now, but this was an official investigation. I would never have thought of lying, whether under oath or not."[9]

When I first began talking to whistleblowers, I found answers like this frustrating. I was looking for a moral justification for their actions, or at least an explanation. But eventually I came to understand that whistleblower narratives are not so much moral justifications as stories about the self. For whistleblowers, the decision to blow the whistle is a choice about the sort of person they are and the one they want to be. It's not a matter of what should be done in the abstract. Sometimes it's not even primarily about the consequences of the choice, although it can be. It is about the personal stakes of keeping quiet. More often than not, what torments whistleblowers is what their decision will reveal about them. They are worried about the state of their soul.

The political scientist Fred Alford spent years interviewing whistleblowers for his book *Whistleblowers: Broken Lives and Organizational Power.* While Alford admired the courage that whistleblowers display, he was struck by how often they turn a moral question about the well-being of others into a moral question about themselves. Even when whistleblowers had acted out of moral principle and felt deep empathy for the victims of wrongdoing, that's not what they talked about. Instead, they talked about themselves: about the values they grew up with, about having to face their children, about the need to hold their heads high. Some whistleblowers said they felt contaminated by their association with wrongdoing. "I just felt so polluted by the whole experience," said a chemist who was fired from his job after he exposed hazardous waste sites.[10]

Alford describes this as "narcissism moralized." Narcissists, he argues, are fixated on their own moral purity. "The narcissist wants to be whole, good, pure and perfect," Alford writes.[11] When narcissists find themselves in organizations that are irredeemably corrupt, they rebel. They push back against the lies, the injustice, and most of all the expectation that they will become like everyone else. This expectation does not just soil them; it makes them angry. Often they become so angry that they will take extraordinary risks to right the wrongs they have seen.

As an example, Alford points to Ron Ridenhour, the American soldier who helped expose the My Lai massacre. Ridenhour felt compassion for the victims, of course, and he was angry at his fellow soldiers for taking part in the massacre. But his deepest rage was directed at the military superiors who sent him and his friends to Vietnam in the first place. "Suddenly he was in a whole new world, a world he didn't want to be in, a world in which he would have to act to purify himself of knowledge he had gained but never asked for," Alford writes.[12] Ridenhour was furious at the military officers who had corrupted his moral innocence.

As much as I admire Alford's work, I believe he is wrong about this. When I talk to whistleblowers, I don't hear narcissism. I hear the ethic of honor and shame. It's true that whistleblowers often talk about themselves, but that's what honor and shame are all about. This is part of what distinguishes the honor ethic from civic virtue, utilitarianism, Kantian deontology, or any number of other moral systems. Honor is about your obligations to yourself. For whistleblowers to talk about themselves is perfectly natural.

"Having honor means being entitled to respect," the philosopher Kwame Anthony Appiah writes.[13] The word "entitled" in his definition is as important as the word "respect." On its own, mere respect is not enough. Respect can be commanded by force or attained by celebrity. But true honor is about being the kind of person who *deserves* the respect they get. It is only by being worthy of respect that honorable people can respect themselves. If they fail, they feel ashamed. This is not wounded narcissism. It is what happens when an honorable person fails to measure up to the honor code.

• • •

To claim that whistleblowers speak the language of honor might sound odd. The very concept of honor strikes some people as anachronistic and others as ridiculous. "The louder he talked of his honor, the faster we counted the spoons," Emerson wrote.[14] It is hard to think about honor without also thinking of pointless duels, vigilante justice, and Don Quixote, tilting at windmills in his rusty armor. Until recently, honor was not even a topic for serious moral philosophy. It was an archaic term whose lost position in moral thought was mourned only by romantics and reactionaries. "Honor occupies about the same place in modern usage as chastity," wrote Peter Berger in a famous essay on its obsolescence. "An individual who claims to have lost it is an object of amusement rather than sympathy."[15]

It is true that the concept of honor no longer has the meaning it once had. Honor was built on a foundation of inequality and rooted in a pre-Enlightenment world of social hierarchies. In the traditional ethic of honor, your duties depended on your social station. The collapse of social hierarchies in the eighteenth century dealt a death blow to the concept of honor, which was already on the decline. In its place, Berger argues, arose the concept of dignity. Whereas in the ethic of honor your worth came from your social station, with dignity your worth came from your status as a human being. Dignity, unlike honor, is universal. It extends to everyone. As the United Nations states in the Universal Declaration of Human Rights, "All human beings are born free and equal in dignity and rights."[16]

Yet concepts rarely just vanish, even when the words that describe them start to seem quaint and old-fashioned. We may not live in a world of French aristocrats or Japanese samurai, but we know what honor means. The concept still makes sense to us. "Our language can be seen as an ancient city," Ludwig

Wittgenstein wrote—a complex maze of twisting streets and archaic constructions spreading out into suburbs, where the houses are uniform and the streets are straight and regular.[17] In Wittgenstein's city, honor is like a crumbling old church that has been renamed and renovated, but where Sunday services are still held.

Many of us still feel the moral force of honor, even if we don't use the word. Take, for example, the story of Franz Gayl, an officer in the US Marines and the whistleblower behind a 2007 investigation by *Wired* magazine.[18] Gayl was suspended after he spoke out about the refusal of the military to provide soldiers in Iraq and Afghanistan with armored vehicles. In Tom Mueller's book *Crisis of Conscience*, Gayl explains that his decision to speak out was simple. *"Das macht man nicht.* What was happening was just wrong, and I couldn't let it happen," he said. "I've fallen short in many things in my life. But on this very important thing, I felt, 'No! I've gotta look myself in the mirror.'"[19]

At the heart of the honor ethic lies the sense of potential self-betrayal articulated by Gayl. Unlike the liberal virtues, which usually emphasize obligations to other people, honor is about the duty to oneself. "I've gotta look myself in the mirror," Gayl says, by which he means, "I have to live up to my own moral ideals." Failure under the scrutiny of one's own moral judgment is what the honorable person fears most. The philosopher Anthony Cunningham describes it this way: "In the face of such failure, he is not the man he wished to be—indeed, the man he took himself to be—and he should loathe this fact, provided he really cared in the first place."[20]

The meaning of modern honor is something like that of personal integrity. Both suggest an allegiance to personal moral ideals. But while integrity is private, honor has a public face. Not only do honorable people need to live up to their principles, but they also need to be *seen* as the kind of people who live up to their principles. If they fail, they are ashamed. John Dean felt this way when he was vilified for his role in the Watergate scandal. "I don't want to see people because I'm embarrassed—even, at times, ashamed—to be who I am, or who they think I am," Dean wrote in his journal. "I understand now that we judge ourselves, to a greater extent than I've ever admitted, through the eyes of others. I know it is difficult for any person to consider himself evil, or greedy, or stupid, since he must live with himself. Yet the mirror of my identity is partly in the eyes of others, and I find I keep checking the mirror to see how I look."[21]

When Peter Berger claimed in 1970 that the ethic of honor had been fading from Western thought for centuries, he was only half right. What happened was not so much a disappearance as a change of address. Honor relocated to the interior of the self. In the older, traditional sense, the honor ethic was largely preoccupied with external appearances. It was about formal manners, saving face, deference to authority, and conformity with social expectations. But that began to change when Western societies began to emphasize the importance of individuality and the value of private, interior experience. This shift allowed honor to become harnessed to moral dissent. As Frank Barrett and Theodore Sarbin have argued, the modern concept of honor is constructed around "an inner self who knows right from wrong, engages in self-appraisal, and struggles against a potentially unsympathetic world."[22]

The prototypical modern struggle over honor involves a self-reflexive conversation between what Barrett and Sarbin call the "self as author" and the "self as actor." When the author passes judgment on the actor, the author needs to feel a measure of pride. Honorable people understand that doing the right thing may come at a personal cost. The world may condemn them, and they may find themselves ostracized and shamed. Framing the struggle often involves an imagined conversation between these two selves: "If I don't do the honor-able thing, I won't be able to live with myself."

As evidence, Barrett and Sarbin cite a study in which forty-five naval officers were asked to relate a story in which they saw the ethic of honor at work. Not a single officer wrote about honor in the traditional sense. They didn't write about sav-ing face, responding to an insult, or maintaining their reputa-tion. Instead, they wrote about staying true to an inner voice despite social or institutional norms that demanded other-wise. One wrote about a commander who had stood up to his superiors and refused to fire an officer he believed in. Another wrote about reporting an instructor he saw strike a student, despite the false denial of the victim. In most of the stories told by the naval officers, acting honorably meant paying a personal cost in order to maintain one's self-respect.

Honor can also lead to terrible acts, of course, especially acts of violence. Some of the worst violence is often directed toward those who break the code of loyalty. What makes the honor ethic important for understanding whistleblowing is not its substance so much as its structure. Whistleblowers take great personal risks to stay true to an inner moral com-pass. This is why Barrett and Sarbin see whistleblowing as the paradigm case of modern honor. Like the rest of us, modern whistleblowers may well believe that all people deserve to be treated with respect. What gives that belief such tremendous power, however, is the sense that failing to speak out about a breach of respect would violate their personal moral code.

The conventional view of whistleblowing is that it is a sim-ple moral choice. Yet the more carefully you listen to whis-tleblowers, the more complicated their actions come to seem. Whistleblowers feel morally obligated to speak out, yet they often feel bad about doing it. Many of them understand they are embarking on a professional suicide mission, yet they feel as if they have no choice but to do it anyway. Some of them feel complicit in the crimes or sins of their organizations and feel ashamed, yet they acknowledge they have played no part in the wrongdoing. Perhaps most troubling of all, many whistleblowers come away from their experience deeply scarred—even if they are vindicated, even if the wrongdoers are punished, even if there is justice for the victims. To understand these puzzles, we must understand the nature of honor.

• • •

A gray day, an empty restaurant, a wary woman sitting across the table from me. She has just hobbled in on crutches. "Sasha," as I will call her, is not sure whether to trust me. A former research study coordinator, Sasha blew the whistle on fraud in a university endocrinology department in California twenty years ago. (I have changed certain potentially identifying details.) The principal investigator was falsifying data and cutting corners, mainly to enroll more subjects into the study. Sasha, who had no medical training and no previous experience in medical research, initially cooperated with the fraud, largely because she thought she was doing patients a favor by getting them into the study. But when she came to understand the potential dangers of the study drug, not to mention the fact that she could be held responsible, she reported the fraud to the department chair. Within a day she was fired.

"I was incredibly naive. I thought I'd report this, and they'd fix it," Sasha tells me. Decades later, she still shows scars from the experience. Her manner is nervous and guarded, and she keeps glancing at the exit. Although Sasha hired a lawyer and forced the endocrinology department to take her back, she was given a low-level position that she found tedious. "I was a pariah. I was a leper," she says. "Nobody would make eye contact." Eventually, she quit the job and moved overseas. The university took no action against the endocrinologist or the department chair.

Several years later, Sasha got a call from an attorney. The Department of Justice was bringing federal fraud charges against the endocrinologist. The attorney said that a teenaged girl in the study had committed suicide. This news shook Sasha. The longer she thought about it, the more obligated she felt to act. "I was going to get justice for this kid," she tells me, her eyes welling with tears. She decided to testify that the endocrinologist had committed fraud. "I wanted justice," she said.

What she didn't anticipate was how viciously the endocrinologist's defense attorneys would attack her credibility when the trial began. With relentless precision, the attorneys revealed deeply personal details about her private life, all of which were made public by a local reporter covering the case. Once again, Sasha felt blindsided. "I blew the whistle on him," she says. "My life should not have been part of that." Of everything that Sasha went through, it was the humiliation of this experience that she found the most painful.

The trial ended with a fraud conviction for the endocrinologist. The administrators who had covered up his fraud were forced to resign. A newspaper columnist called Sasha a hero. To an outsider, it might seem that Sasha came away victorious. But to her it has never felt like much of a victory. Sasha doesn't believe the punishment the endocrinologist received was sufficient, and although decades have passed since the scandal, it is still hard for her to talk about the experience. She is baffled that so many others who knew about the fraud did nothing. "How do you stand by and let these things happen? You go to bed at night. You look at yourself in the mirror. I don't understand." When I mention the article that called her whistleblowing heroic, Sasha gives me a look that suggests I have lost my mind. "I didn't run into a burning building," she says. "I just did what was right, with the naive expectation that others would do the same."

In many ways, this is a story of honor and shame. The reason is not just Sasha's principled dissent, her feelings of self-obligation, her anger at seeing her reputation attacked, or even her sense of vengeance. It is her flat dismissal of the idea that she behaved heroically. This is not false modesty. From outside the ethic of honor, acting with courage despite such grave risks may look like heroism. But from the inside, it is simply what honor demands. You might as well be called a hero for taking care of your children or filling out your income tax forms honestly. As Appiah writes, "An honorable person will often think that what he has done is simply what he had to do."[23]

When whistleblowers are asked why they spoke out, they often reply that they had no choice. They were forced to act; there was no other option. So common are such descriptions that they have a rote, almost formulaic quality. Yet the whistleblowers are clearly describing something deeply felt. Fred Alford calls it a "choiceless choice."[24] The fact that the phrase is self-contradictory doesn't mean that it is nonsensical. By saying "Here I stand, I can do no other," whistleblowers are conveying just how powerful the moral compulsion to act felt to them. Some whistleblowers even speak about their actions with an air of bewilderment, Alford says, as if they had been sent off to fight an angel or a devil. For Alford, it is obvious why whistleblowers use the language of compulsion, especially those who have suffered greatly. To say they had no choice relieves them of some degree of responsibility for an action that may well have ruined their lives.

Václav Havel, the playwright and Soviet-era political dissident who eventually became president of the Czech Republic, explains how it felt for him in his famous essay, "The Power of the Powerless." "You do not become a 'dissident' just because you decide one day to take up this most unusual career," Havel writes. "You are thrown into it by your personal

sense of responsibility, combined with a complex set of external circumstances. You are cast out of the existing structures
and placed in a position of conflict with them. It begins as an
attempt to do your work well and ends with being branded an
enemy of society."[25]

That Sasha simply took the honor code for granted is
understandable. The research oversight system is built on the
assumption that researchers will behave honorably. Institutional Review Boards do not typically monitor clinical investigators or inspect their facilities. Nor do they double-check
reports to make sure investigators are actually doing what
they say. "I will begin by noting that IRBs are not policing bodies, watchdogs or auditing agents," Dr. Robert Levine told the
US Congress in 1998. Levine was a Yale University physician,
a research ethicist and the editor of the ethics journal *IRB*.
"IRBs were established to work collaboratively with investigators," Levine said, "the vast majority of which are altruisti-
cally motivated and intend to do the right thing."[26]

Levine may be right, but with an honor code, altruism and
good intentions are not enough. Researchers must be committed not only to doing the right thing, but also to ensuring
that others do the right thing as well. As Appiah points out,
any kind of morality will tell you that it's wrong to cheat on a
test, steal from the company, or abuse prisoners of war. But it
takes a sense of honor to drive people beyond mere condemnation to insisting that something must be done when people
on their own side betray the code: "It takes a sense of honor to
feel implicated by the acts of others."[27]

• • •

A number of years ago, when my son Crawford was looking
at colleges, we visited a liberal arts college that is very proud
of its honor code. Students pledge not to cheat, and the college takes them at their word; nobody proctors their exams

or runs their papers through a plagiarism detector. As our small group of prospective students and their parents moved slowly through the spreading oaks and gray stone buildings of the campus, a student-guide walking backward explained how the honor code worked. The longer she spoke, the more agitated one of the parents became. First the parent frowned, and then she started shaking her head gravely, and eventually she raised her hand. "Here's what's bothering me about your so-called 'honor code,'" she said. "If you don't have anybody watching the students take their exams, doesn't that mean they have to watch each other? And turn in anybody they see cheating? That's disgraceful. How can an honor code require people to snitch on their friends?"

It was a reasonable question. I can imagine new students at the college wondering the same thing. But when our student-guide tried to answer, she stumbled. First she started down one avenue, then she detoured down another, and eventually she landed on individual conscience as a solution. She said it was up to students to decide for themselves how they felt about turning in someone who had cheated. At this point Crawford leaned over to me and said, "That doesn't sound like an honor code. It sounds more like honor suggestions."

He was right, of course. An honor code is not a recommendation, an aspirational principle, or a rule of thumb. It is a demand for principled adherence. Unless students are morally committed to enforcing it, an honor code won't work. Yet I still felt bad for the student who tried and failed to defend the code, because this aspect of honor can be very jarring for modern sensibilities. Reporting a fellow student for cheating does feel like betrayal. That's part of why whistleblowers feel so tormented. Only when failing to report cheating is a far greater torment will a college honor code be effective. Students must feel as if they are a part of the college; they must feel a deep obligation to the role of the honor code within the life of the college; and they must feel as if a violation of the code represents a moral breach in which they have a personal stake. Some of them might even feel ashamed that it has happened.

"The psychology of shame is at the heart of the psychology of honor," writes Anthony Cunningham.[28] This is why whistleblowers often feel complicit in the crimes of others. Honor and shame are deeply bound up with identity, including collective identity. You can be ashamed of your children. You can be ashamed of your parents. You can be ashamed of your country, your church, your military unit, or your alma mater. If it's part of your identity, you can feel ashamed—as well as pride when it performs well. This is not because your moral purity has been stained, but because you identify with the person or organization behind the shameful actions. As a South Carolinian, I feel deeply ashamed of my state's legacy of racism. I don't feel this way about German war atrocities. I feel appalled and horrified, but not ashamed. These were not my people's crimes.

Shame overlaps with guilt, but the two concepts are different. Guilt is almost exclusively moral. You feel guilty for your crimes and sins. Shame covers a much broader territory. Many of us feel ashamed of failures that have nothing to do with morality—our weight, our clothes, our inability to make a free throw when the game is riding on it. Nor is shame only about what you have done. You can also feel ashamed of things that were done to you or even things that simply happened: a slip of the tongue, a punch in the nose, a rip in the crotch of your pants. Unlike guilt, which is private, shame is fundamentally about exposure. It involves the imagined gaze and judgment of another person. "Shame is a reaction to other people's criticism," the anthropologist Ruth Benedict wrote. "It requires an audience or at least a man's fantasy of an audience. Guilt does not."[29]

You can't escape shame by escaping the audience, of

course. If that were true, you could rid yourself of shame by exiling yourself to a distant place where nobody knew what you had done, like Lord Jim in Patusan. But that would not work any better for an honorable person today than it did for Jim. Shame travels with you. It lives in your head. Once the chip has been installed, it can't be removed. For this reason, an effective honor code doesn't require external surveillance. Those bound by the code can't escape their own judgments, at least not without the aid of alcohol or heavy psychoactive medication. This is one reason why honor codes, such as they are, have traditionally been associated with institutions where surveillance is difficult or expensive, such as medicine and the military. We need soldiers who will act with courage even when no one is watching, and we need doctors who will act with respect and decency even in the privacy of an examining room.

That many whistleblowers identify strongly with the organizations whose corruption they expose is no accident. Daniel Ellsberg was a former US marine. He worked at the Pentagon under Secretary of Defense Robert McNamara. He spent two years in South Vietnam. A sense of complicity drove his decision to give the Pentagon Papers to reporters. "Keeping silent in public about what I had read and heard made me an accomplice," Ellsberg says in the documentary *The Most Dangerous Man in America.* "It was not only they who had all these decisions quiet, hidden from the American public. I had kept them quiet."[30] At some point his silence became unconscionable, and Ellsberg had to separate himself from the wrongdoing. The way he phrases his choice is revealing: "I am not going to be part of this system of lying anymore." It was not just that the Pentagon was doing terrible things; it was that he felt he was implicated in those terrible things if he didn't try to stop them. This is the language of honor.

To outsiders, feeling ashamed of sins that you did not commit might seem like a recipe for irrational self-loathing. "I'm ashamed of what my company did, and I'm ashamed I had to blow the whistle," a whistleblower told Fred Alford. "I'm ashamed for the people I worked with, and I'm ashamed for the people who were hurt by what my company did." When Alford asked him why he felt ashamed when he knew he had done the right thing, he replied, "Because I was part of that world."[31] Self-loathing this may be, but it is not irrational. In the ethic of honor and shame, this explanation makes perfect sense. Honor and shame are not just about what you have done, but about *who you are*. In writing about honor in the old South, historian Bertram Wyatt-Brown said, "One feels recreant not for a particular misdeed but for one's complete existence, a totality of unworthiness because the fault or misconduct fully defines the individual in others' eyes and therefore in one's own."[32]

The watchword of the honor code is sincerity. An honor code cannot easily survive irony or subversion; it would only be a slight overstatement to say that it must be held sacred. Those expected to abide by the code must revere it. The code must also be fair. The force of a code depends on it being revered as much by those at the top of the organization as those at the bottom—not just soldiers, but also generals; not just college students, but also administrators; not just doctors, but also hospital CEOs. The moment when an honor code comes to be seen as something only for suckers and chumps is the moment when it begins to crumble.

• • •

On May 22, 1856, on an otherwise uneventful day in the United States Capitol, a thirty-six-year-old representative from South Carolina named Preston Brooks approached the desk of Charles Sumner, a senator from Massachusetts. After a brief explanation, Brooks proceeded to pummel Sumner mercilessly on the head with a cane. When the cane snapped, Brooks didn't stop. He kept pounding away with the piece of cane he had left. Nor did he stop when Sumner collapsed, bleeding and nearly unconscious. Brooks simply lifted him up by the lapel with one hand and thrashed him with the other. So vicious was the caning that Sumner had to be carried out of the Senate chamber. Three years would pass before he was able to resume his duties.[33]

What triggered the incident was an insult to the honor of Brooks's family. In an oration on the floor of the Senate, Sumner, an abolitionist, had ridiculed several proslavery Democratic senators. One of them, Senator Andrew Butler, was a cousin to Brooks. Sumner had mocked Butler's pretensions of honor and chivalry. He had compared Butler to Don Quixote and called him a mad zealot. He made fun of Butler's speaking ability—"the loose expectoration of his speech"— which was impaired by a facial palsy. Using suggestive sexual metaphors, Sumner said Butler had chosen a mistress "who, though ugly to others, is always lovely to him; though polluted in the sight of the world, is chaste in his sight. I mean the harlot, Slavery. For her, his tongue is always profuse in words." In a summation dripping with sarcasm, Sumner insinuated that Butler was suffering from delusions of grandiosity. "Heroic knight! Exalted Senator! A second Moses come for a second exodus!"

It was an effective speech in service of an admirable cause. It was also a calculated insult, and in the antebellum South, honor demanded that an insult be answered. Failure to respond would mark a man as a coward. Butler was not present for the event, so the responsibility fell to his cousin. Brooks had originally intended to challenge Sumner to a duel, but after consulting with a fellow South Carolinian, he had concluded that duels were intended for gentlemen of equal social standing. As a Northerner, Sumner probably would have refused to duel anyway. Brooks chose to beat him with a lightweight gutta-percha cane of the type often used to train an animal. The caning shocked the Senate, but back home it transformed Brooks into a folk hero. South Carolinians sent him hundreds of new canes, one of which bore the inscription "Hit him again."[34]

Every ethical system has its flaws and weaknesses, and to a modern eye, one of the most deeply troubling features of the honor ethic has always been violence. The demand for respect may sometimes lead to righteous protest and dissent, but it has also fueled honor killings, mafia hits, school shootings, gang wars and family feuds that have festered for generations, not to mention countless brawls in parking lots and bars. In America, the honor ethic is strongest in the South, where the planter class used its code of honor to justify chattel slavery for centuries. Even today, the South is the most violent region of the United States. What fuels Southern violence is not the commission of felonies such as armed robbery, which occur no more often in the South than elsewhere. It is violence in response to insults, slights or other threats to a man's honor.[35]

Ryan Brown, a social psychologist at Rice University, in Texas, has studied the honor characteristics of people in each American state, attempting to understand the lens through which people interpret social interactions. The states least associated with the honor ethic tend to be clustered in the North and the Midwest, especially the Upper Midwest. Minnesota, the state where I now live, ranks near the bottom of the honor scale, with only North Dakota ranking lower. By contrast, the states ranking highest on the honor scale are located mainly in the South and, to a lesser extent, the West. These are the states that experienced a large eighteenth-century migration of Ulster Scots, a people well known for their honor culture. The state that ranked highest on the honor scale was South Carolina.[36]

A set of famous empirical experiments involving honor and violence was conducted by social psychologists at the University of Michigan in the 1990s.[37] The purpose was to see whether Southerners responded differently to insults than Northerners. The psychologists arranged a scenario in which unsuspecting subjects walking down a hallway encountered a stranger, who, unknown to the subjects, was a confederate of the psychologists. As they passed in the hall, the stranger bumped them and muttered "asshole." The difference in responses was striking. Northerners laughed the insult off. Southerners boiled with anger. This difference was not merely evident in their behavior. In Southerners, lab tests showed dramatically higher increases in cortisol and testosterone, chemical markers of stress and aggression.

Unlike dignity, which everyone possesses simply by virtue of being human, honor depends on the respect of others. This is why responses to insults have traditionally been so important in the honor ethic: an attack on someone's reputation cuts to the core of who that person is. It also explains why honor cultures place so much importance on politeness and manners. If an insult can lead to death, injury, or a public caning, you want to be very careful with what you say. In another experiment at the University of Michigan, social psychologists found that when a stranger blocking the hallway was not insulting, Southerners were more courteous to him than Northerners were. I imagine them stepping aside to say, "After you."[38]

Few whistleblowers resort to violence, although I suspect some of them have fantasized about it. More relevant to the whistleblower's crusade is a related feature of honor cultures: vengeance.[39] A thin gray zone separates the driven whistleblower who acts honorably to expose an injustice and the malicious one who just wants payback. Public relations professionals fully understand this; it is partly because revenge is such an understandable motive that organizations intent on discrediting whistleblowers inevitably accuse them of being spiteful and vindictive. To dismiss such accusations as universally wrong would be too easy, of course. Problem employees do exist; many unhappy workers do want to settle old scores. Yet just because a whistleblower is motivated by revenge doesn't mean that her cause is not righteous. Honorable whistleblowers who refuse to back down are often punished so relentlessly for so long that it would be bizarre if they didn't harbor a grudge.

Modern liberals sometimes dismiss vengeance as a primitive, even barbaric sentiment. Yet the fact that revenge is such a popular theme in American movies and novels suggests that even liberals secretly understand its appeal. The outlines of the revenge tale are familiar from classic Westerns: a solitary figure seeks to right a wrong, usually in a lonely landscape where the traditional institutions of justice have failed. Transpose the setting from the Wyoming Territory to an academic health center and you could be describing many research whistleblowers. It wouldn't be surprising if they sounded a lot like the narrator of *True Grit*, Mattie Ross, an obstinate Arkansas Presbyterian who lost her arm at age fourteen on a mission to avenge the murder of her father. If Mattie feels any regrets about killing her father's murderer, it doesn't show in her description of it. "I hurriedly cocked the hammer and pulled the trigger," Mattie explains. "The charge exploded and sent a lead ball of justice, too long delayed, into the criminal head of Tom Chaney."[40]

It is possible, of course, for whistleblowers to act with no thought of revenge. Some people harbor no grudges, have no wish to revisit past wrongs, and are completely unmoved by stories of Old Testament justice. I am not one of those people. Nor, I suspect, are many others who blow the whistle. Why else would a whistleblower battle fruitlessly for years to expose abusive studies that ended long ago, that pose no threat to any living human, and that were conducted by researchers who have since retired or died? Rarely is revenge irrelevant to these battles. It is not that whistleblowers fail to understand how deeply self-destructive the thirst for vengeance can be. It is not that they haven't seen how a destructive cycle of retribution can destroy nations, tribes, and families. But in a world where the usual mechanisms of justice are absent or corrupt, where every effort to right a simple wrong is met with punishment and contempt, time has a way of transforming even the most kindhearted people into avenging angels, determined to smite down their enemies with the hammer fist of justice.

Consider Nancy Olivieri, the hematologist at the University of Toronto's Hospital for Sick Children who famously exposed the dangers of an experimental thalassemia drug manufactured by the drug company Apotex.[41] When Olivieri defied Apotex and published her alarming research results in the *New England Journal of Medicine* in violation of a confidentiality agreement, she was not only fired from her administrative position but forced to endure years of harassment, threats, smears, litigation, and professional marginalization.[42] The fact that the University of Toronto was negotiating an enormous financial donation from Apotex during the scandal no doubt played some part in its craven response.[43] In one notorious incident, a colleague, Gideon Koren, was discovered to be sending anonymous "poison pen" letters aimed at discrediting her.[44]

I have known Nancy Olivieri for over a decade, mainly as a principled supporter of other whistleblowers. Her dark, self-mocking sense of humor makes our conversations easy, although many of them probably couldn't be broadcast uncensored. What is a little hard to reconcile is the gracious, kindhearted person I know with the ferocious street fighter I have only read about, a woman who not only blew the whistle on a deceptive pharmaceutical company but made her adversaries regret bitterly that they retaliated against her. The record suggests that she is a very dangerous enemy. Nancy simply explains that she is Italian.

The Apotex controversy simmered for decades. There were official reports, investigations, lawsuits, dueling newspaper and magazine articles, an academic journal symposium, a controversial nonfiction book, even an episode of *60 Minutes* in which the CEO of Apotex, Barry Sherman, was caught in a lie and called Olivieri "nuts."[45] What separated Olivieri from most other whistleblowers was her relentless determination to make her attackers pay. For every punch she took, Olivieri punched back harder, often with the aid of an attorney. "Honestly, I was just driven by rage—rage that they could do this," Nancy tells me. She freely admits that revenge and accountability were, in part, strong motivators. In fact, she's proud of it. To her, some injustices are worth obsessing over. To those who say that she needs to get over it, Olivieri disagrees. "I guess if you were to tell me that Daniel Ellsberg was kind of over it, I would say, well, there isn't much to Daniel Ellsberg's character."

Organizations typically control whistleblowers with the threat of retaliation. If the tactic were not effective, organizations wouldn't use it. But in some cases it backfires. Instead of intimidating the whistleblower, it motivates them. The more often they are humiliated, the less likely they are to consider a peace offering. The more abuse they face, the more convinced they become that the organization is evil beyond redemption. Every effort to intimidate such whistleblowers simply hardens them in the belief that their enemies can't be trusted. Even if their dissent began as a mission to protect research subjects, that mission eventually fuses with the whistleblowers' determination to vindicate themselves publicly. And so they find themselves locked in a cage match with the organization for years, absorbing blow after brutal blow, convinced that defeat would mean dishonor. These people do not give up easily.

• • •

For many whistleblowers, life is divided into two parts: before and after the event. Whistleblowing changes their lives in an elemental, almost primitive way. Why this is true for those who have suffered brutal retaliation is no mystery. Many whistleblowers lose everything. Their careers end in ruins. They are forced into bankruptcy. Their spouses abandon them. It is as if they awoke one day to find themselves living out the Book of Job: destitute, lonely, bereft of their children, covered in boils. No wonder they descend into a swirling eddy of rancor and self-loathing. Like Job, they struggle to understand why the righteous are persecuted.

Yet some whistleblowers survive their ordeal without life-destroying punishment. Not every whistleblower is escorted out of the building by a security officer. Some people manage to blow the whistle without being fired, demoted, disciplined, or sued. If they file a successful qui tam lawsuit, they may even become rich. Yet many of those same people still emerge from the experience deeply scarred. Their view of the world has been irrevocably altered, like a soldier returning from a combat zone. Often their scars remain unhealed for years, even if they succeed in their mission and find public vindication. Why should this be so?

I put this question to Tom Devine, the legal director of the Government Accountability Project and an attorney who has been helping whistleblowers since the late 1970s. Devine says that many whistleblowers see their decision as a crossroads moment that will reveal what they stand for. Yet at this particular crossroads, both paths lead to damnation. Unable to betray their principles, the whistleblowers feel compelled to betray their organization. "This is their world. This is their environment. This is their community, their culture, and now there's an adversarial relationship with it. And whether they win or lose, it's going to have a long-term impact on them," Devine says. "It's so disruptive of the premises that define your identity, your self-image, who you are."

What makes these ordeals especially hard to endure is their epic duration. Rarely is blowing the whistle a simple, straightforward affair. Often it drags on for years with no finish line on the horizon. "You don't just drop the truth in the hopper," Devine says. "No, it's a marathon process." Nor does the battle end with clear winners and losers. Almost never does David's stone strike Goliath on the forehead and send him crashing to the ground. If an investigative journalist reports damaging information, the organization denies it. If a journalist or regulatory agency demands documents, the organization stonewalls. If there is victory in court, the organization files an appeal. If the whistleblower gets any public vindication, it is often partial and contested in a way that makes it feel incomplete. Many whistleblowers are never able to put the episode behind them, in part because it's never quite clear that the episode is over.

For some people the disruption is even more profound. To become a whistleblower requires a certain measure of idealism. There is a good reason hardened cynics don't blow the whistle: They are convinced that the system is rigged. They feel certain that the reward for blowing the whistle will be a private self-immolation ceremony witnessed only by their gloating enemies. Whistleblowers see the world differently. They believe not just that some actions are so disgraceful that they must be exposed, but that others will be as outraged as they are. Like Martin Luther King Jr, they are convinced that the moral arc of the universe bends toward justice. So when their claims of corruption and cruelty are met with a shrug, not once or twice but every single time, they come away deeply shaken and disoriented. The experience comes as a profound existential collapse, like discovering that your husband of thirty years has been living a secret life with another wife and family in Bridgeport, Connecticut. What do you do when everything you thought you knew about the world is wrong?

Many whistleblowers feel terribly lonely. They become orphans, exiles, castaways. A part of them feels ashamed of their innocence, like the third grader exposed as the only kid in class who didn't know that Santa Claus was really his parents. But alongside that shame is a kind of revulsion at the world that has been revealed to them. How is everyone else capable of working so happily with the knowledge that their organization is corrupt? Are they willfully blind? Alford says that many whistleblowers he interviewed spoke of their coworkers as zombies. "Sometimes they just don't seem human," one whistleblower told him. "I think people must kill a part of themselves to remain part of the system."[46]

· · ·

When Alexander Butterfield left public office, he found himself in a strange kind of purgatory. Democrats distrusted him because he had been part of Nixon's White House. Republicans hated him for betraying Nixon's secret. "I was neither a good guy nor a bad guy. I was an enigma," Butterfield said. Finding a job was difficult. CEOs shied away from him. Exiled from his former friends and colleagues, Butterfield struggled to find a place in the world again. "So, generally speaking, those first ten years for me were not happy," he said. "In fact, it was a fairly miserable period."[47]

Especially painful was that his exile came from behaving honorably. Honor does not demand respect from everyone, but it does demand respect from what Appiah calls an "honor world"—a group of people who acknowledge the same codes of behavior.[48] Respect can be lost, refused, or taken away. And when honorable people no longer have the respect of those in their honor world, they struggle to maintain their self-respect. Some never do. "One has to recapture his self-esteem," Butterfield said. He had to keep reminding himself that he had once been considered good at his job.[49]

For some whistleblowers, this loss of respect is one of the most devastating aspects of their experience. They have spoken out because someone in their honor world has violated the code and they feel morally betrayed. Only when the violation is acknowledged and repaired can the group meet the demands of honor. But when the whistleblowers speak out, the group turns on them. They are seen not just as traitors, but as traitors who must be destroyed so that nobody will believe their accusations. So the whistleblowers are denied precisely what they need to restore their self-respect. They need ratification from their community; what they get instead is exile. They are expelled from the group. They're told, "You're not one of us anymore."

An especially crushing part of this exile is the feeling of betrayal by friends and colleagues, especially friends in a position to help. Sometimes the signs are subtle. Phone calls go unreturned. Invitations dry up. A chilly air descends on casual conversations. It is not uncommon for colleagues to express support in private but refuse to acknowledge the whistleblower in public. Frank Camps was an engineer for Ford who protested the unsafe design of the Pinto, a car that would become notorious for exploding in rear-end collisions. At first the other engineers said, "Go get 'em, we wish we could do it, there goes a man with brass balls." Camps says, "While I had tacit support, I was looking for an honest man to stand with me." No one stepped forward. It wasn't long before his colleagues were given promotions and raises while Camps was frozen out. He said, "Next thing I knew, I didn't have the support anymore."[50]

Allen Jones was an investigator in the Pennsylvania Office of the Inspector General when he discovered that his own office was implicated in pharmaceutical industry corruption. His investigation into the fraud was not welcomed. "Everyone at work looked at me like I was a cobra," Jones said. "I couldn't have been more alone if they put me in the toilet."[51] Eventually, Jones was fired. His debts mounted, and his marriage ended in an acrimonious divorce. Jones moved into a hunting cabin in the woods of central Pennsylvania, where he slept with a gun underneath his pillow. Although Jones eventually won a large qui tam settlement, the experience left him with a sense that the world was broken. When Tom Mueller met Jones years later for his book *Crisis of Conscience,* he found a man who was still stunned that the world had turned on him for doing the right thing. "It is hard to fully trust anyone or anything again," Jones said.[52] Mueller compared him to the driven protagonist of a Greek tragedy, traveling a path foretold by the Fates.

To rebuild an identity in exile demands a kind of resiliency that not everyone has. Rejection is never welcome, of course, but rejection by the people you respect and admire is an especially hard blow, especially if that blow is a punishment for holding principles you assumed that everyone shared. Some whistleblowers try to change jobs, but this can be difficult. Rarely does a reputation for blowing the whistle help anyone find work in their field. More often it makes potential employers wonder if the whistleblower can be trusted. Others move far away or try to vanish into anonymity, as if they had entered a witness protection program.

What whistleblowers require is a competing narrative, or what the philosopher Hilde Lindemann Nelson calls a "counter-story."[53] They need a story that explains what has happened in a way that does not leave them feeling broken and helpless. Ideally, that story will constitute an interpretation of the facts that restores the whistleblower's self-respect and shows them a path toward rebuilding an identity. This can't simply be a private story. It won't work for a whistleblower to construct a story in isolation, like a prisoner in solitary confinement proclaiming his innocence. To be truly effective, the story needs to be ratified by others, preferably a community of people that the whistleblower respects.

The problem is finding that story. The notion of the whistleblower was invented in the 1970s as a way of reframing the Judas story. By turning a story of betrayal into a story of righteous dissent, supporters of whistleblowers sought to construct a counter-story that would morally affirm the actions of people like Daniel Ellsberg, Frank Serpico, and Ron Ridenhour. But their efforts were only partially successful. They may have succeeded in rehabilitating Judas, but the result was a version of the David and Goliath story, a narrative in which whistleblowers not only triumph over long odds to defeat the mighty organization but are celebrated for remaining true to their consciences. The problem is that this story doesn't track reality, at least not for many whistleblowers. Most whistleblowers are not celebrated, and they don't defeat Goliath. What these people need is a story of moral affirmation that can restore their self-respect in the absence of any external reward.

Alexander Butterfield eventually moved from Washington, DC, to California, where nobody knew who he was and few people cared about Watergate. "They'd say, Water-what?" Butterfield said. Anonymity suited him. He built a new career in business and earned a master's degree in history from the University of California, San Diego. He didn't let the world destroy him. By reminding himself that he was a good person who had earned the respect of others in the past, he managed to hang onto his self-esteem. He even took some pleasure in the way things turned out. "I rather enjoy looking the jerks, the people I know put selfish personal interests before probity, squarely in the eye," he said. "I feel that I have so much more than they do."[54]

That Butterfield managed to tell himself a story of moral affirmation doesn't mean that he was unconcerned with competing stories. In a 1989 interview, Butterfield admitted that he was bothered by a Trivial Pursuit question that identified him as the man who revealed the existence of the Watergate tapes. To Butterfield, this way of describing his role suggested that he had intended to bring down Nixon, or even that he had gone to investigators with the damning information. Neither of these things were correct. It troubled Butterfield that people might think his motives were sinister, unpatriotic, or self-aggrandizing when he simply told the truth. When the interviewer asked Butterfield how he would prefer the answer to be phrased, Butterfield's answer was revealing. He said he would rather be remembered as "one of the few people who answered questions honestly."[55]

CHAPTER 2

Tuskegee

It is a July evening in 2016, at the Viva Goa restaurant in San Francisco, and I am sitting across from a silver-haired gentleman named Peter Buxtun. We've just ordered our meal when a loud thud sounds from across the room. Buxtun, who is nearly eighty, leaps up from the table and rushes over to help a dazed-looking woman sprawled on the floor. "Did you hit your head?" Buxtun asks. "Are you okay?" When she doesn't answer right away, Buxtun switches to German. Yes, she is fine, although very embarrassed; apparently, she had misjudged the location of her seat and sat down in empty space.

As Buxtun is helping the woman to her feet, a waiter pushes his way between them to fill her water glass. The waiter is intent on pretending that nothing unusual had taken place, even though it has been only seconds since the woman had crashed to the floor. When Buxtun returns to our table, he is still shaking his head, baffled by the waiter's behavior. This reaction is not uncharacteristic of Buxtun. Despite his easy laugh and genial manner, he has the air of a man who fears the world is populated by blockheads and scoundrels.

In 1972, Buxtun exposed the most notorious medical research scandal in American history. For forty years, the US Public Health Service had deceived and exploited hundreds of poor Black men with syphilis near Tuskegee, Alabama, using free meals and burial insurance to lure them into an experiment in which they would receive no treatment for a potentially deadly disease. Very few employees of the health service apart from Buxtun saw anything wrong with this. Only when Associated Press reporter Jean Heller wrote about the abuse, using documents provided by Buxtun, did the Tuskegee study eventually end. Buxtun's revelations triggered Senate hearings, a federal inquiry, a class-action lawsuit, and, in concert with several other research scandals of the period, a broad-reaching set of federal guidelines and institutional structures intended to protect the subjects of medical research.[1]

It would be difficult to name a figure in the history of American medical ethics whose actions have been more consequential than Buxtun's. Yet most ethicists have never heard of him, and many accounts of the Tuskegee scandal do not even mention his name. Buxtun did not appear in Jean Heller's 1972 exposé, nor was he mentioned in the first major scholarly article about the scandal, written in 1978 by Harvard historian Allan M. Brandt.[2] In the well-known play (and later, film) based on the scandal, *Miss Evers' Boys*, Buxtun is completely absent. His name is rarely uttered along with the other notable whistleblowers of his era, such as Daniel Ellsberg and Frank Serpico. If the role played by Buxtun in exposing the scandal is at all familiar, it is largely because of James H. Jones's influential 1981 history of the Tuskegee study, *Bad Blood*, and Wellesley College historian Susan Reverby's 2009 book, *Examining Tuskegee*.[34]

Included in *Bad Blood* is a photo of Buxtun as a bearded

young man in 1973, posing next to Senator Ted Kennedy. For many years that photo—plus the knowledge that Buxtun lived in San Francisco during the 1960s—had placed a certain image of him in my head. If asked to describe it, I would have mentioned radical politics, psychedelic drugs, and maybe the Grateful Dead. Nothing could be less accurate. Buxtun is a life-long Republican, a member of the National Rifle Association, and a collector of vintage weapons. When I told him about a recent visit I had made to the City Lights bookshop, famous as the home of San Francisco's Beat poetry scene in the 1950s, he replied, "Sometimes I like to go there and ask to see their military history section." Buxtun left the Public Health Service in 1968, moving on to law school and then to a career in investments, but he has lived in the same Telegraph Hill apartment for more than fifty years. In front of a large bay window overlooking San Francisco Bay is a set of German aviation binoculars mounted on a tripod. The walls of his apartment are lined with bookshelves, including one shelf devoted to books he keeps solely for their names. One is titled *The Romance of the Gas Industry*.

Buxtun is an exceptional figure, and not just because he is among the few people to blow the whistle on a major research scandal. Even among whistleblowers, Buxtun is an outlier. He did not witness any wrongdoing firsthand. He worked thousands of miles away from the place where the scandal occurred. Before the Tuskegee experiment became public, he had never met any of its victims. He was not punished for blowing the whistle, nor is he tormented by memories of the experience. Perhaps most unusual of all is Buxtun's relative success in exposing the study. With the possible exception of the Nazi concentration camp experiments, the Tuskegee syphilis experiment is probably the only example of abusive medical research that most Americans could name.

Yet even those who can name the Tuskegee study often

misunderstand it. In medical school ethics courses, the Tuskegee syphilis experiment is taught as part cautionary tale, part reformist success story; a case study in exploitation and racism that changed the face of medical research. The reality is more complicated. It took Buxtun seven years to expose the experiment. The public health establishment fought him at every turn. When the study was finally exposed, the federal government resisted paying for medical treatment for the victims. Another twenty-five years passed before the government apologized. The reforms that were initiated in the wake of the Tuskegee experiment have not kept research subjects safe; the United States continues to see outrageous research abuses. In fact, if not for a unique set of historical circumstances combined with Buxtun's bullheaded tenacity, it is unlikely that Buxtun's whistle would have ever been heard.

· · ·

Buxtun never planned to work for the Public Health Service. Raised on a ranch in Oregon, he had enlisted in the army and trained as a psychiatric social worker after he finished a political science degree at the University of Oregon. In 1965, he was doing graduate work in history when he saw a job flier. The health service was funding a venereal disease program in San Francisco. Buxtun says, "I found this thing and thought: San Francisco, working in VD control? What a stitch!"

Soon he had become a venereal disease tracker. "A typical day would be, come in, look in your mail slot to see if you had some other people's names," Buxtun says. "Charlie Jones, met in a gay bar by another gay guy, and they had gay sex, the other guy had syphilis. Okay, chase this guy down. How do you find the guy? Well, there are a lot of ways to do it, and we had some of the resources that a typical detective in a police department would get—reverse directories and things like that." Once Buxtun had tracked his subject down—

sometimes in a flophouse, sometimes in one of the city's better neighborhoods—he would persuade the person to be tested. Those who tested positive were treated effectively with penicillin. "Men could get a sore that would scare the hell out of you," Buxtun says. "One of them looked like a dog had taken a bite out of a weenie."

One day in the coffee room in the fall of 1965, Buxtun overheard a coworker talking about a syphilis patient in Alabama. "The family knew that he was really ill, that something was really wrong," Buxtun says. "He was plainly insane, had symptoms, and for some reason they took him some distance away to a doctor they knew of." The doctor diagnosed tertiary syphilis (the later stages of infection, which can damage the central nervous system) and gave the man a shot of penicillin. But when Public Health Service officials found out, they got very upset. The doctor, unaware of the Tuskegee study, had treated a research subject who was not supposed to be treated.

The next day Buxtun was on the phone with someone at the Communicable Disease Center (now the Centers for Disease Control, the CDC). "I said, 'Hey, what do you have on this Tuskegee study?' He said, 'Oh, I've got a lot on it. What do you want?' I said, 'Send me everything.' Damned if I didn't get— and I've still got it—a brown manila envelope." It had about ten reports of what were called roundups—the occasions when the subjects were found and brought in for examination. What Buxtun read about the Tuskegee study in that envelope contradicted everything that he'd been advising doctors to do with a syphilis patient. "You treat him. You don't let him get back out in society and infect someone else," Buxtun says. Yet in Tuskegee, the researchers were simply following patients to see what would happen if they went without therapy. "It was an autopsy-oriented study," Buxtun says. "They wanted these guys dead on a pathology table."

The research subjects were all Black men in Macon

County, Alabama, many of them sharecroppers. The purpose of the study was signaled in the title: "Tuskegee Study of Untreated Syphilis in the Negro Male."[5] Nearly four hundred subjects had syphilis and another two hundred or so served as healthy controls. The syphilitic men were never told they had an infectious disease, only "bad blood," nor were they offered any treatment apart from tonics and pills, such as aspirin for aches and pains. Many subjects underwent painful lumbar punctures (spinal taps) to determine whether the infection had spread to the nervous system. The researchers persuaded them to enroll in the study by giving them free meals and minor remedies and by promising to pay their burial expenses in exchange for permission to autopsy their bodies. When the Tuskegee study began in 1932, treatment for syphilis involved a lengthy, toxic course of arsenic-based therapy. By 1943, however, the disease was easily curable with penicillin. The consequences of untreated syphilis are summed up on a yellow matchbook that Buxtun and his colleagues used to distribute in bars and bathhouses: "Blindness, heart injury, insanity, death."

Buxtun took the roundup reports with him to the city library. "I wanted to look up German war crimes proceedings," he says. Buxtun had come to America as an infant in 1937, the son of a Jewish Czech father and a Catholic Austrian mother. He knew that the "Doctors' Trial" in Nuremberg, in which German physicians were indicted for experimenting on concentration camp prisoners—seven physicians were executed—had led to the modern code of research ethics. The very first principle of the Nuremberg Code states, "The voluntary consent of the human subject is absolutely essential." The code also directs researchers to protect subjects from disability, injury, or death, no matter how remote the possibility. Buxtun remembers, "It was toward the end of the evening in that library downtown, and I thought: I've got to do something."

The first thing he did was prepare a report on the Tuskegee study. "I directly compared the work of the CDC in Atlanta, in Tuskegee, to what the Nazis had done," Buxtun says. He showed the report to his boss and said he planned to send it to William Brown, the head of the Venereal Disease Section of the Public Health Service. He recalls his boss saying, "When they come to fire you, or do whatever they're going to do, forget my name. I've got a wife and a couple of kids. I want to keep my job."

It is unclear whether Brown ever read that report, but he certainly read a letter Buxtun sent him in November 1966. "Have any of the men been told the nature of this study?" Buxtun asked. "In other words, are untreated syphilitics still being followed for autopsy?" Brown drafted a reply assuring Buxtun that the subjects were volunteers who were "completely free to leave the study at any time." But he apparently never sent it and instead decided to talk to Buxtun in person.

"To my surprise, I got orders to go to Atlanta, from Dr. Brown and company," Buxtun says. "I was being called on the carpet, and they thought from the high position that they had that they were going to correct an errant employee. Maybe I was an alcoholic, or a lunatic of some sort." The March 1967 summons to Atlanta coincided with an annual conference for health care workers specializing in venereal disease. When Buxtun arrived at the conference hall, however, he didn't get the welcome he was expecting. "I went up to the place where they were handing out the badges," Buxtun says. "And they said, 'You're not on the list.' What do you mean I'm not on the list?" Buxtun laughs as he remembers the confrontation. "They said, well, there's this chair over there, about 40 feet away, and there's probably a magazine around. You should sit there on that chair and read a magazine or two until the conference is over." Buxtun thought, "Until the conference is over? The hell with that! So, I waited until no one was looking and I walked in."

After the first session, Buxtun returned to his chair. "So these stern-looking bureaucrats come out," he says. They led him to a meeting room with a large, dark wooden table. "All these guys came in and sat at one end of the table, so I went a little way down the table, sat down, and put my things down," Buxtun says. They were sitting right in front of the American flag and the flag of the Public Health Service. The leader of the group was Brown, who turned out to be a "mousy little bureaucrat," according to Buxtun. The real enemy in the room was John Cutler, an assistant surgeon general and venereal disease specialist who was deeply involved in the Tuskegee study. "He was bursting with rage," Buxtun remembers. "He couldn't wait for the door to be shut to that meeting room."

"That guy pinned my ears back," Buxtun says. "He proceeded to give me a tongue-lashing. 'See here, young man. This is serious work we are doing. You are talking about harm to these Black sharecroppers? This is something they are doing as volunteers.'" Buxtun responded by reading from one of Cutler's own reports, which stated clearly that the subjects would never have agreed to the study without the "suasion" of burial expenses. Buxtun remembers Cutler saying, "I didn't write that! I didn't write that! It must have been written by one of my colleagues!" At that point, Buxtun says, everyone in the room began to look nervous.

• • •

In 1967, when Buxtun traveled to Atlanta, clinical research was still a relatively small-scale affair, conducted largely in academic medical centers and government institutions. Twenty years had passed since the introduction of the first modern code of research ethics, the Nuremberg Code, which was developed in response to Nazi medical atrocities. The Nuremberg Code was followed by the Declaration of Helsinki, a more detailed code of ethics adopted by the World Medical Association in 1964. Both codes were largely aspirational, and medical research still took place with little formal oversight. The conventional view of the Nuremberg Code was described by Yale University ethicist Jay Katz: "It was a good code for barbarians but an unnecessary code for ordinary physician-scientists."[6]

A major challenge to that view came in 1963, when ordinary physician-scientists at the Jewish Chronic Disease Hospital in New York injected twenty-two elderly, debilitated patients with live, cultured cancer cells.[7] The injections were part of a study designed to understand the immune response, and the researcher in charge was Dr. Chester Southam, a respected oncologist and immunologist. But the elderly subjects in the study never knew they were being injected with cancer. Nor did they have any reason to suspect that the injections weren't part of their clinical care. Many of them were Holocaust survivors whose first language was Yiddish. So alarming was Southam's study that three younger physicians had refused to cooperate. Avir Kagan, David Leichter, and Perry Fersko were all Jewish and had lost family members in the Holocaust; Leichter was himself a Holocaust survivor. When Southam's study went ahead anyway, they submitted a letter of resignation to the hospital board. A board member filed a lawsuit against the hospital, igniting a public furor.

Three years later came yet another challenge. In 1966, Harvard University anesthesiologist Henry Beecher published a bombshell article in the *New England Journal of Medicine*, "Ethics and Clinical Research."[8] Beecher described twenty-two studies in which investigators had "risked the health or the life of their subjects" without telling them of the dangers or getting their permission. None of the studies were secret. They had all been published in medical journals, many of them quite prestigious. Nor were they taken from the distant past. All the studies had occurred in the postwar period. One was Southam's experiment at the Jewish Chronic Disease Hospital. Another was the deliberate infection of mentally disabled children with hepatitis at the Willowbrook State School.

A year after Beecher's article appeared, the English physician Maurice Pappworth published *Human Guinea Pigs*, an even more disturbing catalog of abusive experiments that included many conducted on children and mentally incompetent adults.[9] Unlike Beecher, Pappworth named the culpable researchers and laid out a prosecutorial case against them. In one noteworthy example, Pappworth described how researchers in New York had bored holes in the skulls of patients, implanted "trephine buttons," and subjected the patients to an array of procedures in order to see their effects on cerebral circulation: cutaneous pain, carbon dioxide inhalation, neck vein compression, nicotinic and alcohol injections. At the root of these ethical abuses, Pappworth argued, was the "maniacal impulse" among academic physicians to publish research papers in order to get promotion and tenure.

Many academic physicians disagreed. It wasn't just that they were unhappy to see their dirty laundry aired in public. Many of them didn't think the laundry was dirty. As the Harvard University immunologist Geoffrey Edsall wrote a few years later, academic physicians thought that their public image was being unfairly transformed from heroic Arrowsmiths to predatory Elmer Gantrys, pious con men preying on the vulnerable.[10] The backlash against the Jewish Chronic Disease Hospital scandal had come only a year after the Kefauver hearings of 1962 aired concerns about the devastating effects of thalidomide. Public opinion about medical research was turning. It didn't take a sophisticated appreciation of public relations to realize that something needed to be done.

What many academic physicians feared most was the threat of outside interference.[11] None of them wanted their research to be formally regulated. They wanted as little outside scrutiny as possible. Far better than regulation would be

an in-house mechanism for protecting human subjects, perhaps a peer review committee over which they could exert
some measure of control. In July 1966, the academic physicians got their wish. William Stewart, the surgeon general,
issued new Public Health Service guidelines stating that
clinical researchers with federal funding must submit their
research to a "committee of institutional associates."[12] The
new guidelines defused the threat of formal regulation. The
in-house committees that Stewart put into place would eventually become the Institutional Review Board system that
oversees medical research today.

Yet outsiders were still interested in the ethics of medical
research, especially theologians and moral philosophers. In
1967, the American Academy of Arts and Sciences ran the first
of two conferences on the topic "Ethical Aspects of Experimentation with Human Subjects." The most important paper
to emerge from these conferences came from Hans Jonas, a
German-born Jewish philosopher who had fought the Nazis
in World War II and whose mother died in Auschwitz. Jonas
put his finger on the critical aspect of human experimentation
that distinguishes it from most other human interactions.
Human research subjects do not exercise agency; they are
the object of actions by others. "What is wrong with making a
person an experimental subject is not so much that we make
him thereby a means," Jonas wrote, "as that we make him a
thing—a passive thing merely to be acted on."[13] The danger
for clinical researchers, Jonas thought, is that of coming to
see their subjects purely as experimental material. When the
Tuskegee study was exposed five years later, the reality of that
danger became disturbingly clear.

• • •

Buxtun heard nothing more from William Brown after his
summons to Atlanta. In November 1968, seven months after

the assassination of Martin Luther King Jr, Buxtun wrote to Brown once again, this time pointing out the political volatility of the study. "The group is 100% negro. This in itself is political dynamite and subject to wild journalistic misinterpretation," Buxtun wrote.[14] Brown didn't respond. Instead, in the spring of 1969, he convened a "blue-ribbon" panel, this time with experts from outside the Public Health Service. But even the blue-ribbon panel decided against stopping the study.

Although Buxtun was unaware of it, he was not the only person to find the Tuskegee study objectionable. Over the decades, a handful of others had protested. Some were physicians at other universities who learned about the study from lectures or journal articles, such as Count Gibson, of the Medical College of Virginia, and Irwin Schatz, of Henry Ford Hospital in Detroit.[15] Another was a Public Health Service employee: Bill Jenkins, an epidemiologist and one of the first African Americans to work for the CDC. Jenkins went so far as to organize opposition to the study and attempt to alert the press.[16] Yet none of the dissenters had the staying power of Buxtun, who for seven years simply refused to let the issue die.

By the early 1970s, Buxtun had left the Public Health Service for law school but was still living in San Francisco. Among his circle of friends was a group of women who had been at Stanford together, one of whom was Edith Lederer. She would later become the Associated Press correspondent for the United Nations, but in 1972 she was only six months into her first job as an AP reporter. Buxtun started telling her and some of her journalist friends about the Tuskegee study. "I remember one night, a bunch of us went to a pizza place, and two of these reporters were right across the table from me." He gave them his pitch. "This one guy looked at me, put his pizza down, and said, 'Look pal, we deal with the news all the time. Give us a break. We just want to have a pizza.'"

A month later at a dinner party, he tried Lederer again.

"That night she listened," Buxtun says. He recalls her saying, "What? Black people? All of them Black?" Lederer asked Buxtun if he had any documentation. "We'd had dinner already so I said come on, hop in my car, and I'll show you." Lederer can still remember her reaction to those documents. "I was horrified," she says. Buxtun says Lederer was sitting on the couch in his apartment. "She kept looking and looking and finally she said, 'Can I borrow this and xerox it?' And I said, 'I wish you would!'"

By 1972, seven years had passed since Buxtun first objected to the Tuskegee study. During that period, the civil rights landscape had shifted considerably. In 1968, Martin Luther King Jr. had been assassinated. Protests and riots had engulfed Chicago, Baltimore, Washington, DC, Kansas City, and other cities. Earlier that year, police in Orangeburg, South Carolina, home of South Carolina State University, had opened fire on Black protestors, killing three and injuring another twenty-eight. George Wallace, the race-baiting governor of Alabama, had run for president on the American Independent Party ticket in 1968, campaigning on a platform supporting racial segregation. Wallace carried five states in the Deep South. In 1972, he was running again.

Lederer took the documents to her bureau chief, who wanted to pursue the story but thought that Lederer was too inexperienced to report it herself. He allowed Lederer to decide which reporter should replace her. Lederer sent the material to Jean Heller, an investigative reporter in the Washington office. On July 25, 1972, Heller's article appeared in the *Washington Star* and on the AP wire service. When it was reprinted the next day in the *New York Times*, it carried the headline, "Syphilis Victims in U.S. Study Went Untreated for 40 Years."[17]

"It just blew the story wide open," Buxtun says. Not only did the Tuskegee revelations shatter the popular image of doctors as honorable professionals, but they also confirmed the Black community's worst fears about institutionalized medical racism. That such a study could be sponsored by the federal government was bad enough. That it could continue in plain sight for four decades—the results published openly in medical journals with little objection or comment—was stunning. Before Tuskegee, many Americans thought that only Nazi doctors needed formal oversight. After Tuskegee, it was impossible to believe that the honor and good intentions of doctors were enough.

• • •

Jim Jones, the historian and author of *Bad Blood,* can remember exactly where he was when the news of the Tuskegee experiment broke. An Arkansan by birth and a historian by training, Jones was heading east from Indiana to start a fellowship in bioethics and history of medicine at Harvard. He was planning to do research on the social hygiene movement. "I was literally driving across the country from Bloomington to Cambridge to start that fellowship and Jean Heller broke the story," Jones says. "I spent the night on the road and decided that I was not going to work on social hygiene; I was going to try to find out more about Tuskegee."

It wasn't the first time Jones had heard about the Tuskegee experiment. "I'm the guy who should have been the whistleblower but was too stupid," he says. Jones first came across documents about the Tuskegee experiment when he was doing research in the National Archives as part of his doctoral dissertation on Alfred Kinsey. "I'm slogging through, dutiful graduate student that I am, four hundred and twenty-something letter boxes of stuff at the archives, and everything that I see deals either with prophylaxis or the treatment of syphilis. And then I come across this stuff on this untreated syphilis program in Macon County in Alabama," Jones says.

He was not shocked. He had come across other nontherapeutic human experiments during his research. But Jones had just assumed that this one had ended in the 1930s. "It wasn't until Jean Heller wrote that story that I thought, 'Shit, it's still going on!'"

A few days later Jones learned that the Department of Justice had ordered the National Archives to sequester its material about Tuskegee while they investigated. Knowing how the Nixon administration operated, Jones worried that the Department of Justice would deep-six all the Tuskegee documents and cover up the scandal. A friend at the National Archives told him that the documents had already been moved to a federal records center, an enormous repository to which the public is not generally allowed access. But Jones persuaded his friend to bend the rules and let him see the documents. Soon Jones had four letter boxes on the origins of the Tuskegee experiment. It wasn't long before he had contacted Fred Gray, the attorney representing the Tuskegee victims. "The next day he was in my home," Jones says. "He spent a few hours leafing through the material and he was like a guy in heaven."

Jones says his first introduction to Peter Buxtun came through Buxtun's letters, which Jones found in the CDC archives. "I think it's impossible to read those letters without understanding that you're in the presence of an extraordinary person," Jones says. "He wasn't a high-ranking person. He was a spear carrier." He calls Buxtun the person who says the king is naked. "For him to have been as clear-sighted, as morally focused, as persistent as he was, and to speak truth to power—I thought it was extraordinary, and I wanted to meet him, and when I did meet him, everything that I saw fit with the guy I thought I knew."

When Jones and Buxtun met in person, Jones was working for the National Endowment for the Humanities in Washington, DC. "My wife and I were then living on East Dupont Circle. We had two kids and two floors of a townhouse, a small brownstone," he says. Jones and Buxtun hit it off immediately and spent a long day talking about the Tuskegee study. But at five o'clock the next morning Jones was jolted awake by someone throwing pebbles at his window. "So, I get up and look down and Peter's standing in the street," Jones says. "Let's go horseback riding!" Buxtun shouted. "I've got this friend down in Charlottesville and she's got horses. Grab the kids and Linda and let's do some horseback riding!" Jones told Buxtun to go back to bed.

Decades later, sitting on a couch in his Telegraph Hill apartment, Buxtun still has the irrepressible enthusiasm of a much younger man. There is a mischievous, almost boyish quality to his manner, especially when he shows me his antique weapons or the fake ammunition on his desk: a shotgun cartridge flashlight, a mortar shell cocktail shaker. When I admire the yellow matchbook that the Public Health Service used to distribute ("San Francisco's VD problem is your problem. Help solve it."), Buxtun jumps up from the couch and tells me to wait. A few minutes later he emerges with an identical matchbook and cheerfully presents it to me as a gift.

As gracious and funny as Buxtun is, our conversation would be easier if I were better at keeping him on topic. While all my questions are about Tuskegee, his answers veer away toward things he finds more interesting: political outrages, the presidential race, a story from his army days about a soldier who thought he was a werewolf. Buxtun is eager to share his opinions, but he is not inclined toward introspection. What he relishes is tweaking the conventional wisdom. When he gets rolling with an especially delicious story, his smile widens and turns a little crooked. A devious look appears in his eye. I suspect he has always been a contrarian. According to Susan Reverby, the author of *Examining Tuskegee*, the reports Buxtun wrote for the Public Health Service were "likely to quote from *Conservative Viewpoint* on Washington politics or from Dante's *Inferno*."[18] Reverby says, "He must have driven his supervisor nuts."

Yet Buxtun identified closely with the Public Health Service and felt proud of what it did. This was why he was so upset by the Tuskegee experiments. "Look, we took our work seriously," he says. "I had a business card from the San Francisco Department of Public Health, and it was very valuable to me. I did not have a badge. I did not have a gun." The exploitation of poor Black men in Alabama felt like a betrayal of the PHS mission. When I ask Buxtun whether he had any fears or doubts about opposing his superiors, he replies no, none at all. I believe him. Buxtun does not seem like a man who is easily intimidated. "Did it ever occur to you that you might be wrong?" I ask. Buxtun seems puzzled by the question. "No, I had the evidence," he says.

This is not to suggest that he was naive. Buxtun was well aware that his efforts to stop the Tuskegee study might backfire on him. "You bet I thought about having to find another job, perhaps in another city and probably outside of government," Buxtun tells me. "Make no mistake, my confrontation with the CDC aristocracy was intended to get rid of me. They knew it, and I knew it."

If Buxtun was ever afflicted by feelings of disloyalty to the Public Health Service, he doesn't show them now. Nor is he plagued by guilt, shame, or thoughts of self-recrimination. Remarkably, he seems to hold little malice toward those who disagreed with him or refused to help. When I ask what kept him so intent on exposing this scandal for so many years, he replies, "I'm a child of the Holocaust." Buxtun says he is often asked, "Why does a white guy like you have anything to do with Black people you've never met working in a field in Macon County, Alabama?" He says his reply is simple. "Because it shouldn't be happening. Because it's happened elsewhere. This is Nazi medicine."

• • •

Buxtun was never punished for blowing the whistle. That fact alone sets him apart from most whistleblowers, many of whom face vicious retaliation. In 2010, scholars at the University of Chicago and the University of Toronto studied 216 cases of corporate fraud. They found that in more than 82 percent of cases with named employees who reported fraud, those employees were fired, quit under duress, or were punished in some other way. Many never worked again. The scholars concluded, "Not only is honest behavior not rewarded by the market, but it is penalized. Why employers prefer loyal employees to honest ones is an interesting question that deserves separate study."[19]

This pattern is consistent across a whole array of organizations, both public and private: engineering firms, banks, military units, government agencies, and hospitals. Even nurses who speak up about dangers to patients are often punished. One study found that 28 percent of nurses who reported misconduct were formally reprimanded, and every single nurse surveyed suffered some kind of informal retaliation, such as ostracism or pressure to resign. Ten percent were asked to see a psychiatrist.[20]

Although I have been unable to find similar studies of whistleblowers in clinical research, there is little reason to think the results would be much different. One of the most demoralizing recent assessments of medical whistleblowing came from a Harvard study of twenty-six people who had exposed fraud and corruption in pharmaceutical companies using qui tam lawsuits. The purpose of qui tam lawsuits is to encourage whistleblowers by allowing them to collect a share of the resulting financial settlement. Many of the whistleblowers eventually collected millions of dollars, but few felt that it was worth the personal devastation. Often they had been asked to take extraordinary risks, such as smuggling files out of the company or wearing a wire to meetings, yet federal investigators treated them with suspicion, as if they were complicit in the crimes. Nearly half of the whistleblowers experienced stress-related illnesses, and more than 30 percent were financially ruined.[21]

Of course, most people who learn about organizational wrongdoing don't blow the whistle. When those people are asked why they remained silent, they usually give one of two reasons.[22] The first is that nobody would listen. The second is fear of retribution. For decades, findings such as these have guided reformers who want to encourage whistleblowers. The Whistleblower Protection Act of 1989, for example, made it a federal offense for government agencies to retaliate against government employees who report things such as waste, mismanagement, and violations of the law.

Yet many witnesses to wrongdoing in medical research are academic physicians, many of them protected by tenure. These physicians can't be fired, at least not easily. They are skilled, high-status professionals with a measure of financial stability to fall back on if things go bad. Yet still they usually remain silent. Most of us understand intuitively how difficult it is to defy authority or break from a group, especially a close-knit group, even if doing so presents no real danger at all. The true horror of My Lai and Jonestown—or, for that matter, any number of college hazing scandals—is not that the shame of going along with the group is unimaginable, but that we can imagine it all too well.

In 2012, a team of social psychologists in Amsterdam, Padua, and Palo Alto designed an unusual study of research whistleblowing based on Stanley Milgram's famous obedience experiments at Yale in the early 1960s.[23] In an elaborately constructed sham scenario, Milgram's subjects were ordered to administer what they believed to be dangerous electrical shocks to unwitting people. The subjects weren't enthusiastic about obeying; in the films Milgram made of the experiment, you can see the subjects sweating, trembling, and repeatedly protesting as they increased the "shocks" to the highest voltage. Yet in the end, faced with a conflict between the demands of their conscience and those of a man in a white coat, more than 65 percent obeyed the man in the white coat.[24]

In the new version, the social psychologists wanted to see whether people would blow the whistle on an obviously dangerous experiment. They arranged for groups of Dutch university students to be approached by a stern, formally dressed "scientist" (actually an actor) who wanted help recruiting volunteers for a study of sensory deprivation. The scientist told the students that his experimental subjects would be isolated and unable to see or hear anything for an extended period. An earlier pilot study had gone badly; the traumatized subjects had hallucinated, panicked, and lost their ability to think rationally. Two of the six subjects had begged to have the experiment stopped, the scientist explained, but stopping it would have ruined his data. Now the scientist was repeating the experiment with younger subjects, whose brains were even more sensitive to the traumatic effects of sensory deprivation. He wanted the Dutch students to help him by recommending the experiment by email to their acquaintances and friends. Those who agreed to help were instructed to write a statement using at least two of the words "exciting," "incredible," "great," or "superb."

This study was designed to make it as easy as possible for the subjects to refuse to cooperate and blow the whistle to an oversight committee. The "scientist" left the room so that no subject would have to confront an authority figure, and the subjects were given plenty of time to consider their decisions. In addition, the subjects were told that the university's research committee was still deciding whether to approve the study. The students were all given a form encouraging them to register any ethical objections, which they could submit anonymously.

When a group of subjects was asked to predict how they would handle such a scenario, virtually none of the subjects could imagine themselves cooperating. More than 96 percent said they would disobey the scientist or blow the whistle to the research committee or both. But when a matched group of subjects was placed in a room with the fake scientist, the overwhelming majority complied. More than three-quarters of the students wrote a statement intended to recruit their friends and acquaintances into the dangerous study, and only one in ten blew the whistle to the research committee.

What accounts for this alarming result? Certainly not fear of retribution or a sense of futility. Subjects could register their dissent confidentially, and there was no reason for them to believe that the research committee would ignore their concerns. Nor was it anything about the subjects as individuals. Personality tests could detect no differences between those who resisted authority and those who obeyed. According to the psychologists who designed the study, the explanation is simply the one that Milgram laid out decades ago: in most situations, we simply do what is expected of us by people we see as legitimate authorities. Milgram called this surrender of autonomy the "agentic state."

The phrase sounds like something from *The Manchurian Candidate*, but there is nothing sinister about it. In most social situations, we expect that someone will be in charge—a host at a dinner party, a flight attendant on a plane, an usher at the theater. In such situations, we naturally do as the authority tells us. The problem, of course, comes when a legitimate authority figure asks us to do something cruel or dishonest. According to Milgram, we often try to weasel out of such conflicts by imagining ourselves as mere instruments for the wishes of the authority. Adolf Eichmann claimed he was just following orders; today, we're more likely to excuse ourselves by saying, "Above my pay grade" or "Not my circus, not my monkeys." A version of this response came through in the whistleblowing experiment. The subjects who cooperated tried to deflect responsibility to the fake scientist, while the rare subjects who blew the whistle did so precisely because they felt personally implicated.

Of course, in actual cases where research subjects are mistreated, the potential whistleblowers are often highly trained, knowledgeable adults with medical expertise, not students listening to a research presentation for the first time. Like Buxtun, they have the chance to do their own background reading, ask tough questions, and talk to colleagues. Rarely is there a single moment of decision, as there was for the students; potential whistleblowers usually have months or even years to ponder their choices. Yet many of them still fail to act.

As alarming as Milgram's findings were, they also suggested a solution. By manipulating study conditions, Milgram found that he could tip the scales away from obedience and toward the demands of conscience. Diminishing the prestige of the authority figure helped—getting rid of the scientist's lab coat, for instance, or moving the experiment from Yale to a nearby community building. So did bringing the victim into the same room as the person administering the shocks, so that the screams and protests by the victim became more personal. But the most profound changes came when Milgram placed dissenting confederates in the room. If the "scientist" was accompanied by a second "scientist" who objected to the shocks, not a single subject was willing to continue administering them. And if a person was placed at a table with two others who refused to administer shocks, that person was emboldened to resist as well. In other words, people were far

more likely to follow their conscience if they didn't feel so isolated and alone in their dissent.

Inspired by Milgram's findings, researchers at the University of Michigan designed a different sociological experiment
in the late 1970s to examine "encounters with unjust authority."[25] Like the Milgram experiment, this one involved deception: a group of strangers were brought into a room under
the guise of participating in a focus group. In fact, what the
researchers really wanted to know was how the group would
react to the knowledge that they were being manipulated for
a devious, unjust purpose. At the beginning of the session, the
group was led to believe that the purpose of the focus group
was market research. Over time, however, it became evident
that the real purpose was to gather video testimony that the
leaders would later manipulate to help an oil company punish an innocent man. The results of the experiment confirmed
what Milgram might have predicted. Out of the thirty-three
"focus groups," twenty-five refused to cooperate. Unlike Milgram's study of individuals, which largely revealed obedience
to unjust authority, this study of groups revealed rebellion.

Set against this background of psychological research,
Buxtun's action looks even more extraordinary. In many
whistleblowing stories, what initially looks like an act of individual defiance is actually a story of group cooperation. Whistleblowers are often backed by a group of friends, colleagues,
or fellow travelers. This was not true of Buxtun. He acted
alone—not just in the beginning, but for seven years. "Once
Peter gets something in his head, he's going to pursue it and
give it 100 percent," Jim Jones told me. That Buxtun persisted
so long and eventually succeeded without the help of like-
minded colleagues sets him apart from even the most determined crusaders.

Yet it's also important to note the social factors that made
it more likely that Buxtun would resist authority. He was not a

doctor, so he had not been trained to see senior doctors as his superiors. Nor was he committed to a career in public health. He lived some 2,000 miles from Macon County, Alabama, and the authority figures he answered to in San Francisco were not involved in the Tuskegee study. By the time Buxtun met Brown and Cutler, he had already committed himself deeply to dissent. He never saw the Tuskegee doctors as legitimate authorities and he never surrendered his moral agency to them.

●●●

Most muckraking journalism, even if it is very good, vanishes from public consciousness soon after it appears. Jean Heller's story about the Tuskegee syphilis study was different. Her story ignited a spark that has never really gone out, largely because of the civil rights movement. The civil rights struggles of the 1960s made it possible to see the Tuskegee experiment not just as a single episode of medical wrongdoing but as part of a deeply entrenched pattern of racial discrimination and abuse. The memory of Tuskegee has become a potent symbol of medical racism, a specter that haunts Black patients to this day.

More than any other scandal, the exposure of the Tuskegee experiment triggered major reforms in the oversight of research. In the spring of 1973, a Senate subcommittee chaired by Ted Kennedy held hearings on human experimentation. Those hearings led to the establishment of the National Commission for the Protection of Human Subjects of Biomedical and Behavioral Research, a group of scholars in ethics and medicine that went on to produce the influential Belmont Report. A year later, President Nixon signed the National Research Act of 1974, a piece of legislation that eventually produced three long-lasting institutional reforms: first, the so-called Common Rule, a set of federal guidelines aimed at protecting subjects in federally sponsored research;

second, the federal Office for the Protection from Research Risks (now called the Office for Human Research Protection); and third, the enshrinement of Institutional Review Boards— what the surgeon general called a "committee of institutional associates" in 1966—as the primary oversight bodies for medical research.

It would be a mistake to minimize the importance of these reforms. They represented a major step forward. But it would be a bigger mistake to see the exposure of the Tuskegee experiment as an unmitigated success story. Despite the public outrage over Tuskegee, many public health physicians insisted they were being unjustly persecuted. "There was nothing in the experiment that was unethical or unscientific," declared John Heller, a former director of the Tuskegee study.[26] Others insisted—wrongly—that the subjects had never been prevented from seeking treatment for syphilis. Some of the physicians involved in the study defended it for decades afterward. The federal government didn't even apologize to the victims of the Tuskegee study until 1997, when most of them were dead.

Nor were any of the physicians responsible for the study sanctioned. Just the opposite, in fact: some of them went on to receive honors and awards. The American Sexually Transmitted Diseases Association named its lifetime achievement award after Thomas Parran, the surgeon general and venereal disease specialist who oversaw part of the study, while the University of Pittsburgh, where Parran had served as dean, placed Parran's name on its Graduate School of Public Health.[27] John Cutler, the doctor who pinned Peter Buxtun's ears back in Atlanta, became a department head and acting dean at the University of Pittsburgh. When Cutler died in 2003, Pittsburgh established a lectureship in his honor.[28] (Under pressure, these honors and tributes have now been withdrawn or quietly retired.)

Despite a torrent of negative publicity, the CDC resisted providing medical care for the Tuskegee subjects for eight months while it debated administrative questions. Even more contentious was the issue of financial compensation for the subjects. A class-action suit filed in July 1973 asked for $3 million in compensation for each man or his heirs. But when the case was settled in November of 1974, it was for only a fraction of that amount. Surviving subjects in the syphilis arm of the trial got $37,500; if a subject was dead, his heirs got $15,000.[29] Fifty years after the Tuskegee experiment, the United States remains the only country in the developed world that does not guarantee payment for the medical care of injured research subjects.[30]

Peter Buxtun was invited to testify at the 1973 Senate hearings. As usual, he pulled no punches. "I felt that what was being done was very close to murder," he told the subcommittee.[31] What Buxtun remembers most about his testimony, however, is not what he said but an interruption while he was speaking. "Suddenly the door popped open, and two men ran in," he says. The men approached Senator Kennedy, and the three of them murmured to one another for what seemed like a very long time. "I'm feeling kind of stupid. I'm halfway through a sentence," Buxtun says. Eventually, Buxtun was permitted to finish his testimony. When he returned to his seat, the woman sitting next to him leaned over and whispered, "Haldeman, Ehrlichman and Dean have resigned."

Many whistleblowers find it hard to let go of their bitterness. Buxtun seems remarkably free of rancor. "I've moved on," he says. "A lot of good things have happened." The only figure in the Tuskegee scandal he harbors any resentment toward is Cutler, the man who gave him a tongue-lashing in Atlanta and remained unrepentant for decades. In 2010, the historian Susan Reverby revealed that Cutler had also directed Public Health Service experiments in Guatemala in the 1940s,

in which researchers intentionally gave syphilis and gonorrhea to soldiers, prisoners, and mentally ill patients.[32] In one
especially grisly episode, Cutler dripped gonorrheal pus into
the eyes, urethra, and rectum of a dying, mentally ill woman.[33]
"He's my villain for all of this," Buxtun says of Cutler. "I can see
Dr. Mengele saluting this guy."

Unlike many whistleblowers, Buxtun does not struggle to
understand his experience. While he was never celebrated for
his actions in the way that other whistleblowers of his time
were, his story fits the standard whistleblowing narrative.
Just as David felled Goliath with five smooth stones, Buxtun brought down the Public Health Service with his brown
manila folder. It may have taken seven years of single-minded
perseverance, but his efforts were vindicated by public opinion and the actions of the federal government. It has always
been possible for Buxtun to tell his story with a clear, satisfying ending. That story may be partial and incomplete, but it
ends with an upward curve.

If Buxtun carries any resentment about his relative anonymity, he hides it well. "I don't want to be embarrassed by an
oversupply of compliments," he says. "I am who I am. There's
nothing to try to change, up or down." I tell him I was gratified
to see he had recently been given a Freedom of Information
prize by a journalism association in Northern California. Buxtun replies that he was not the only person honored that night.
Then he adds, "Another recipient was arrested the following
week for public corruption and gun trafficking."

CHAPTER 3

Willowbrook

Mike Wilkins looks like a different person every time I see him. In photos from the 1970s, with his long hair, blue jeans, and droopy mustache, Wilkins reminds me of Cheech and Chong. When we first met in person in 2019, the years had transformed him into a kindly midwestern grandfather with a buzz cut and a brown cardigan. In late October of 2020, as Wilkins walks down the steps of his house in Kansas City, he's a dead ringer for Santa Claus, minus the round belly and merry elves. "This is my protest beard," Wilkins says. The object of his protest is Donald Trump, whose bid for reelection is only four days away. A billowing white beard suits Wilkins nicely in his retirement. "It's gravitas, but it's also a little bit disorderly and unpredictable," he says. "Walt Whitman. Leo Tolstoy. Frederick Douglass." He pauses. "Or Santa Claus." He says if he still has the beard a year from now, he'll put on the red suit and ring a bell for the Salvation Army.

We are standing in front of the handsome, two-story brick

house in the Union Hill neighborhood of Kansas City, where Mike and his wife, Jody, live. Two rocking chairs sit on the porch. On the wall is a white peace sign. Most mornings, if the weather permits, Wilkins takes a walk to The Scout, a statue of a Native American man who peers down from his horse onto the city. This morning I'm here to join him on the walk. I've also brought along a box of books and papers that Wilkins loaned me when he visited Minneapolis a year ago. Most of them are about the Willowbrook State School for intellectually disabled children in New York, the site of the infamous Willowbrook hepatitis study. Wilkins worked there as a physician in the early 1970s.

Like medicine, law, and hard-boiled detective fiction, the field of bioethics is built on cases. Willowbrook and Tuskegee, Quinlan and Cowart, Baby K, Baby L, Baby Fae. Introduced in the standard bioethics seminars, these cases are equal parts thought experiment, cautionary tale, and New Testament parable. When I teach them, my mind drifts back to Sunday School: the prodigal son, the widow's mite, the low, droning hum of an air-conditioning unit. I have become so numb to the repetition of these cases that I thought nothing could change the way I saw them. Yet because of Mike Wilkins, that's exactly what happened with Willowbrook.

The Willowbrook hepatitis study first came to public attention when Henry Beecher published his famous 1966 article "Ethics and Clinical Research" in the *New England Journal of Medicine*. The Willowbrook study was "Example 16." Researchers had intentionally infected "mentally defective" children with the hepatitis virus in an institution where hepatitis was endemic. The parents had given consent, but it was unclear whether they were told of the hazards involved. Citing the research guidelines of the World Medical Association, Beecher wrote, "There is no right to risk an injury to one person for the benefit of others."[1]

Whenever the Willowbrook case is debated, discussion turns to the matter of intent. Most of us recoil at the idea of deliberately infecting someone with a serious disease. What complicates the case were the dire conditions at Willowbrook. So crowded and unsanitary was the school that many children contracted hepatitis anyway, research study or not. If hepatitis was virtually inevitable, why should it matter if the children were infected intentionally? At least the subjects in the hepatitis study were housed in a separate research unit where they could be monitored more carefully.

Such is the usual introduction to Willowbrook: abstract, clinical, matter-of-fact. You can almost hear the low murmurs and coughs at an IRB meeting as the case is discussed around a conference table. Risk-benefit ratio, vulnerable populations, adverse events, informed consent. If you want to bleed a case dry of all human feeling, dissect it with the sterilized instruments of research ethics. Spend an hour or two talking like this and you might even forget that the research subjects were, in Beecher's phrase, "mentally defective children."

Forgetting that is difficult after watching *Willowbrook: The Last Great Disgrace,* a 1972 documentary report about the Willowbrook State School.[2] I can still remember when I saw it for the first time. It was in the fall of 2012. Lyle, my youngest daughter, had just turned eleven. In the early minutes of the film, a youthful investigative reporter named Geraldo Rivera stands in front of a Willowbrook building. "I first heard of this big place with the pretty sounding name because of a call I received from a member of the Willowbrook staff, a Dr. Michael Wilkins," Rivera says. "Dr. Wilkins had just been fired for urging parents of Willowbrook children to demand better conditions." Soon the scene switches to Wilkins himself, sitting on a couch and looking different yet again in his white shirt and striped necktie. Speaking in a soft voice, Wilkins tells Rivera exactly what the children of Willowbrook endure. "Their life is just hours and hours of endless nothing to do, no one to talk to, no expectations, just an endless life of misery and filth."

No description can really do justice to the images in the film. Naked children sit moaning on the floor. Many of them are restrained by straitjackets. At mealtimes, an attendant uses a wooden spoon to shove a gray, grits-like paste into their mouths. Some children simply rock back and forth in crowded, dimly lit rooms, their eyes rolling back in their heads. The images look like something Hieronymus Bosch might have envisioned when he painted *Fall of the Damned into Hell*. Never had I imagined anything this obscene when I discussed the Willowbrook hepatitis study with my students. The thought of my own children in circumstances like these almost made me physically ill. I have seen *Willowbrook: The Last Great Disgrace* at least a dozen times now. The shock has faded with time, but I've never been able to think of the hepatitis study in the same way.

Wilkins and I set off on our walk, both of us wearing COVID masks. He has recently retired from clinical practice as a wound care specialist at the VA Medical Center in Kansas City. If I hadn't known about his history at Willowbrook, I would never have picked him out as a doctor. For one thing, he is far too modest. Wilkins talks cheerfully about his shortcomings and failures without a trace of defensiveness. Nor is he as jaded as most doctors I know. Medicine has not left him with the hard, protective exoskeleton that most doctors start to grow somewhere around their third year of medical school. He has spent his entire career caring for the poor and marginalized, yet I can't detect a hint of sanctimony or self-righteousness about him. He seems remarkably unguarded and vulnerable. It is as if he has decided to open himself up to the world and keep no secrets. He is almost impossible to dislike.

Wilkins has lived most of his life in this city. He grew up in

Des Moines, Iowa, where his mother was a secretary for Standard Oil and his father worked in the Iowa employment security office. Mike was a middle child with a younger brother, an older sister, and an older half brother by his father's first marriage who visited in the summers. The family moved to Kansas City after Mike's freshman year in high school. Both of his parents were alcoholics; Wilkins says his father lost at least one job because of his drinking. Yet Wilkins says they were both wonderful, loving parents. "You could set us up as a typical alcoholic family, and I was the emblematic 'good boy,'" Wilkins says. "I'm the altar boy, I get good grades, and I study hard." Wilkins earned his tuition at his Catholic high school by cutting grass. He loved serving mass at the Little Sisters of the Poor, going room to room with the priest to bring communion to the residents. When Wilkins enrolled at Rockhurst College, a Jesuit liberal arts college in Kansas City, he majored in philosophy.

In the field of bioethics, Willowbrook is synonymous with the hepatitis study, but Wilkins has always seen his work there as a civil rights struggle. He can still remember the first Black person he ever talked to, Dorsey Holly, a maintenance man for the Kansas City parks department. Wilkins had a summer job in high school maintaining the tennis courts, and the two would talk every afternoon under a shade tree. In college Wilkins joined the Congress of Racial Equality, the pioneering civil rights organization founded in Chicago by James Farmer. It was also in college that Wilkins became disillusioned with the church. Wilkins remembers his shock at overhearing a respected priest make anti-Semitic comments to another priest as they were driving to church. Over time, he began to resent being forced by the college to go to mass. Wilkins says that one day after taking communion at a mandatory mass he kept the host in his mouth. After church, as a gesture of protest, he threw it on the grass outside in front of his friends.

To Wilkins, the purpose of the struggle at Willowbrook was to convince others to see mentally disabled people as fellow human beings. *Willowbrook: The Last Great Disgrace* represented a turning point in that struggle. Not only did the film expose the brutalizing way in which the children there were treated; it also showed how intellectually disabled children could thrive when they were treated with love and humanity. One of the most moving moments in the film is an interview with Bernard Carabello, a young man with cerebral palsy who had been at Willowbrook for eighteen years. His keen intelligence is obvious, yet he had been denied an education. Wilkins says he recognized Carabello's potential immediately. "I totally saw him for being a genius the first time I saw him," Wilkins says. Carabello would go on to found the first self-advocacy organization for the disabled in the country and become a disability ombudsman for the state of New York. In 2020 he was awarded an honorary doctorate from the City University of New York, Staten Island.

Before I saw *Willowbrook: The Last Great Disgrace*, I had always seen the Willowbrook study as an abstract puzzle about the nature of responsibility. Is there any moral difference between doing harm and allowing harm to occur? Could a researcher be blamed for deliberately infecting a subject with hepatitis if the subject was likely to get hepatitis anyway? After I watched the film, the nature of the problem changed dramatically. Now I wanted to know what kind of person could go into a place like Willowbrook and see it as a research laboratory rather than a crime scene. The natural human response to such horrific conditions is to feel sickened or maybe to cry. Yet that was not the response of most of the doctors who worked there. Somehow, they had been trained to see things differently. Not only did they tolerate Willowbrook, they propped it up and exploited it.

Mike Wilkins was a different kind of doctor. He didn't go

into Willowbrook as a naive innocent. He took a job there precisely because he suspected that disabled children were being mistreated. Nor was he alone. Wilkins was part of a tight group of radical health care workers with a social mission who remain close friends to this day. That group helped spark a series of events that eventually led to the closure of Willowbrook. The struggle at Willowbrook has clearly left Wilkins wounded, but the wounds didn't come from blowing the whistle. In some ways, Wilkins says, exposing Willowbrook to the world was his salvation.

• • •

Diana McCourt's daughter, Nina, was ten years old in 1971 when she was enrolled in the Willowbrook hepatitis program. Nina was autistic and profoundly disabled, and McCourt was desperate for help with her care. "I just couldn't take care of her in the situation I had," McCourt says. Diana and her husband, Malachy, had two younger children and no money. "We didn't have any services, so I could never take my other children out because of her reaction to going outside," McCourt says. "She would just scream." The Willowbrook authorities told her they had no space available. The school had a long waiting list and there was only one way to jump the queue: enroll Nina in a hepatitis study.

In the beginning, McCourt wasn't worried. She had been told that Nina would be well taken care of and that the study was safe. There was even a special research unit where she would be housed. But her feelings changed once she started visiting Nina. "We weren't allowed to go back where the rooms were," McCourt says. "They would bring her out, and she was really in terrible condition. They were evidently giving her a psychotropic drug that she was allergic to. She was all breaking out in hives." McCourt began demanding that Nina be moved to one of the children's wards, and eventually the administration complied. McCourt says Nina was in the research unit for about four months.

The principal researcher behind the Willowbrook hepatitis program was Saul Krugman, a pediatric infectious disease specialist at New York University. Krugman was on his way to becoming one of the most celebrated pediatricians of his generation. He was chair of his department at NYU. He would soon be elected president of the American Academy of Pediatrics, as well as to membership in the American Academy of Arts and Sciences and the Institute of Medicine. Krugman would eventually win one of medicine's highest honors, the Mary Woodard Lasker Public Service Award, for his contributions to the development of the hepatitis B vaccine.[3] But in April 1972, three months after Rivera aired television footage of conditions at Willowbrook, over 150 protesters tried to disrupt a ceremony in Atlantic City where Krugman was being honored by the American College of Medicine.[4] Those protests were among the first signs that public opinion about Krugman was changing.

The hepatitis study that Beecher called "Example 16" was part of a long-standing hepatitis research program that Krugman started at Willowbrook in 1956.[5] Infectious diseases were a major problem at the school, many of them the result of overcrowding and poor sanitation. When Krugman started his research program, he discovered that many children had shigella, respiratory infections, and intestinal parasites. But the most worrying problem at Willowbrook was hepatitis, an infection of the liver. Hepatitis typically results in diarrhea, abdominal pain, jaundice, and nausea. Most children at Willowbrook seemed to get a mild version of the disease, but hepatitis can be lethal. In poor nations, where sewage often contaminates the water supply, outbreaks of hepatitis A have sickened and killed thousands of people.

Although hepatitis was not well understood in the 1950s,

it was believed that there were at least two types of hepatitis: infectious hepatitis, a milder illness transmitted by the fecal-oral route, and serum hepatitis, a more serious illness that was transmitted through the exchange of blood or bodily fluids. These two forms are now known as hepatitis A and B, respectively. Hepatitis A is the illness we usually associate with poor sanitation and food poisoning; hepatitis B is the illness we usually associate with dirty syringes and unsafe sex. One of Krugman's primary aims at Willowbrook was to understand the natural history of hepatitis—how it was transmitted, its clinical course over time, and the possible differences between the two forms.

A more urgent question was whether medical intervention could protect people from getting hepatitis. Earlier research had suggested that people could get short-term protection from a gamma globulin (a type of antibody) produced in the blood of people who had already been infected with hepatitis. Krugman wondered if gamma globulin might also provide them with longer-term protection. To test this hypothesis, Krugman gave gamma globulin injections to several groups of newly admitted children and followed them for up to two months. Then he compared their rates of infection with that of control groups—similar children who had not been given gamma globulin. The children who had not gotten the gamma globulin injections were much more likely to get hepatitis than the children who had gotten the injection. Just as Krugman had hoped, gamma globulin was very good at protecting children from infection.[6]

If Krugman had stopped at that point, there is a good chance that protesters wouldn't have interrupted his 1972 award ceremony. If he had set into motion a plan to give gamma globulin to all the residents of Willowbrook, they might even have celebrated his accomplishment. But that's not what Krugman did. Instead, he went on to test gamma globulin and another preventive intervention by deliberately infecting disabled children with hepatitis. And he didn't stop with hepatitis A, the milder illness. He also infected children with hepatitis B.

In one study to test whether gamma globulin protected children from infectious hepatitis, or hepatitis A, Krugman fed the children what is commonly referred to as a "fecal milkshake"—chocolate milk contaminated with feces collected from other students.[7] This was the study Beecher later referred to as Example 16. Krugman defended the study by claiming that most of the children would have become infected anyway, but that claim appears to have been exaggerated.[8] A more recent estimate has put the figure somewhere between 30 and 53 percent.[9]

Even harder to defend are some of the studies of serum hepatitis—hepatitis B—that Krugman began conducting in the mid-1960s.[10] In one study, Krugman deliberately injected children with hepatitis B in order to test a proto-vaccine (a heat-treated serum).[11] Hepatitis B infection is much more dangerous than hepatitis A; in the early 1950s, three research subjects who were injected with hepatitis B in federal penitentiaries died.[12] Hepatitis B infection can also lead to chronic hepatitis, resulting in cirrhosis and liver cancer and death. These injections could not be defended with the claim that the subjects would have gotten the illness anyway; the form of hepatitis endemic at Willowbrook was not hepatitis B. As Krugman himself wrote in 1986, "During the course of our epidemiologic survey in 1955, all of the evidence indicated that the endemic disease was so-called infectious or type A hepatitis, an infection that spread via the fecal-oral route."[13]

Whether the consent given by parents was truly informed and voluntary is a matter of some debate. Krugman claimed that his team gave detailed, in-person presentations to the parents. The written consent form he gave to parents was approved by a research oversight body at NYU. Yet that written form was brief and misleading. It obscured the fact that the researchers would infect the children deliberately. And it didn't tell parents of the risks of the study; it only mentioned the potential benefits. In fact, it made the study sound like a preventive intervention, not a research protocol.[14]

To Diana McCourt, consenting to Krugman's research didn't feel like a freely considered choice. It felt like a decision driven by her awful circumstances. Either she could sign Nina up, skip the queue, and have Nina placed in what she believed to be a safe living space, or she could place her on a long waiting list and continue to struggle with her at home. "So, it was a forced decision, really," McCourt says. She was desperate and exhausted to the point of despair. Krugman exploited her desperation. "If you have no choice and you're given an awful choice, I guess you take the awful choice."

In the end, what makes Krugman's studies indefensible is that they could have easily been carried out on fully informed, consenting adults. Hepatitis is not a disease limited to children. Krugman might have recruited the competent adults employed at Willowbrook, including the physicians, many of whom were exposed to hepatitis in the course of their work. Instead, Krugman picked one of the most vulnerable populations imaginable: institutionalized, disabled children. Diana McCourt remembers attending a meeting at New York University where Krugman tried to defend his study. "That was kind of an awakening for me," she says. McCourt says her husband later asked one of the researchers, "Why don't you use chimpanzees instead?" And the researcher replied, "They're too expensive."

Wilkins has complicated feelings about Krugman's work. After he was fired from Willowbrook, Wilkins criticized the ethics of Krugman's study in a debate at New York Medical College. "They were misleading the people who were signing their kids up, and that was what our parents were vocal about," he says. Yet those studies were far from the worst thing about Willowbrook. The children were living in unspeakably squalid conditions. The wards were so understaffed that the children could barely be washed and fed. Krugman's studies may have been exploitative, but they exploited institutional conditions so neglectful and abusive that they should never have been permitted to exist. Wilkins says, "The place was a shit hole to begin with."

. . .

Wilkins first saw the massive brick buildings of Willowbrook from a car window on a cloudy day. "It was like something out of a horror movie," he says. Wilkins was doing a rotating internship with the US Public Health Service Hospital in Staten Island. The head of pediatrics had taken a group of interns to see Willowbrook patients who had unusual congenital anomalies. As soon as Wilkins saw those buildings, he thought of "Pilgrim's Progress," a two-part article by Morton Hunt in the *New Yorker*.[15] It was set at Pilgrim State Hospital, an old, asylum-style psychiatric institution in Brentwood, New York. In 1961, when Hunt's article was published, Pilgrim was the largest psychiatric institution in the world. Wilkins hadn't realized that institutional warehouses like Pilgrim still existed.

Wilkins had joined the Public Health Service after medical school. The military had started drafting doctors, and the Public Health Service looked like a good alternative to Vietnam. In one of the boxes of papers that Wilkins gave me is a Public Health Service memorandum that suggests how he fit into the culture of the organization. Written on official US government letterhead, the memorandum has the subject header "Proper Grooming and Dress." The author is Philip L. Spencer MD, the associate director for ambulatory care. "When you were in my office yesterday I noted that you had only partially corrected your grooming deficiencies," Spencer wrote. "Your mustache still hung down over your lower lip with even longer droopy corners and your hair considerably exceeded the regulation three inches." Spencer ordered Wilkins to correct his "grooming deficiencies" within three days or he would have them corrected by the barber.

In Staten Island, Wilkins and a group of radical health care workers had formed a group called the Fanon Collective, named after Frantz Fanon, the psychiatrist and political philosopher from Martinique who wrote *The Wretched of the Earth* and *Black Skin, White Masks*. One member of the group, David McLanahan, had gone to Vietnam as a medical student and published photos of napalmed children.[16] Another member, Bill Bronston, was a conscientious objector and activist who had been fired from his psychiatric residency in Topeka, Kansas, after organizing a union.[17] Members of the Fanon Collective were marching on picket lines, organizing nurses and social workers, starting day care centers, and providing medical care to the Black Panthers. When Wilkins saw Willowbrook, he saw a new problem for the Fanon Collective to tackle. He decided to apply for a job.

Over the years I've asked a lot of doctors what drew them to medicine. Wilkins may be the only one who has ever answered with a novel. "I read *Of Human Bondage* by Somerset Maugham," he says. Based partly on Maugham's own life, the novel is about an orphaned, disabled young man named Philip Carey who abandons an artistic career to become a doctor. Wilkins remembers contemplating his future in college while working in an especially uninspiring office job: "I just did the math and said, What kind of job am I going to get? I could work in an office like these people, and just drink cups of coffee, and go downhill morally or whatever—like, you know, sell stuff." Medicine seemed like a calling that could fulfill his humanitarian impulses. Wilkins took his first science class in his third year of college and was admitted to medical school at the University of Missouri.

Medical school was a cold shower. Wilkins found the culture repressive and shockingly racist. "The one Black guy in our class flunked out in his first year for dating a white girl," he says. It didn't help that Wilkins was struggling academically. Everyone else in his class had studied biology for years, and Wilkins had never even looked through a microscope. "I damn near flunked out my first two years," he says. His worst subject was embryology. Wilkins despised the professor. "I remember thinking if I just did one thing and choked him to death, that would be the best thing I might ever do in my life."

In his final year of medical school, Wilkins did an obstetrics rotation with a resident named Gary Robinson. Robinson had just delivered the baby of a sixteen-year-old Black girl from the Missouri bootheel and he was sewing up her episiotomy without any local anesthesia. The girl was crying in pain. Wilkins says Robinson stood up, took off his mask, and yelled at her, "Shut the fuck up!" Wilkins asked him why he didn't give the girl anesthesia. Robinson turned and said, "You shut up too." After that incident, Robinson harassed Wilkins unmercifully. "He'd say, 'Wilkins, you stupid shit,' you know, on rounds," Wilkins says. "In my yearbook it said, 'Gary Robinson's favorite medical student' or something like that." Wilkins joined the Public Health Service at the end of the year, grateful to escape medical school.

Wilkins was assigned to Building 6 at Willowbrook and given a cramped, windowless office under the stairs, like Harry Potter's tiny bedroom at the Dursley house. Despite what he had read in the *New Yorker*, nothing really prepared Wilkins for his first day. "This is not what I thought I would be doing," he thought. "Why did I decide to do this?" Building 6 housed 280 children on four wards. The children, who were called "inmates," slept in a large, barracks-like space with seventy cots lined up 2 feet apart. If one of them had a mild illness or a behavioral issue, that child was confined to a locked isolation room with a mattress on the floor. When the children needed to be cleaned, staff members hosed them down as they stood over a drain hole in front of the toilets. There were no medical treatment plans. Wilkins says, "If you come out of a hospital that's a real hospital—and you're really treating patients and discharging them and they're going to get better—and then you go there, it's just a culture shock."

The defining feature of the institution was the small wire baskets hanging on the wall, about the size of a bicycle basket, in which the children kept all their belongings. "You've heard about Mother Teresa and her nuns. They had to carry all their possessions in one little bucket. Same thing for these kids," Wilkins says. Each basket could hold only two changes of clothes and maybe a toy. This became a problem if a child was incontinent. According to Wilkins, "You could dirty up clothes twice, you know, and then you're naked for the rest of the day." Because Willowbrook was so short-staffed, the meals were prepared by residents, working boys and girls who would grind the food into mush. A harried staff member would feed the children with a long wooden spoon as they sat at a table, their mouths open wide. Wilkins says they reminded him of baby birds.

The range of disabilities spanned a broad spectrum. One child was a savant who liked to ask people their birthday and tell them the day of the week it fell on. Another was a sculptor. "This kid would say, 'Silver paper, Dr. Wilkins, silver paper!'" Wilkins says. Wilkins would bring in big rolls of aluminum foil that the child would model into, say, the Verrazzano Bridge. Children with milder disabilities lived upstairs, while the more severely disabled children were housed on the first floor. Many of the children on the first floor were unable to walk or speak, and sometimes they developed disturbing behavioral

issues from being institutionalized. "They would see somebody having a bowel movement, and they would want to eat
it," Wilkins says. "You know, really bizarre shit." When the
children got out of control, staff members would drug them
with Thorazine or Mellaril. "We were by far the biggest consumer of psychotropic drugs on Staten Island," Wilkins says.
"I mean, huge amounts."

Because the doors to the wards were locked, parents were
unaware of the grim conditions that their children faced.
Wilkins says, "The families were told, 'Look, you know, they're
calm and fine back there, but if a stranger comes in they'll all
be upset, and it's not good for them. We will bring your child
to you.' So we would dress the kid up and bring them to the
anteroom off beside the front door." Like Diana and Malachy
McCourt, many parents were desperate for help. Often, they
had been told that their children would be happier around
other children like themselves.

Working with Wilkins at Willowbrook was his friend Bill
Bronston, the de facto leader of the Fanon Collective and an
experienced organizer. Their plan was to reform Willowbrook
into something resembling a humane institution. "When we
went to Willowbrook we were really good revolutionaries,"
Wilkins says. "We were thinking we would organize the workers." But the workers had no interest in being organized. They
were just trying to survive the day-to-day grind of a miserable job. Wilkins could sympathize with their plight. "I mean, I
can't imagine that. I feel bad for myself," he says. "What about
them? They had to work there their whole life."

The two men had even worse luck with doctors. "The
medical staff hated us," Wilkins says. For many of them Willowbrook was a last-resort job, and they weren't about to complain. "If you're going to be a monk, you're going to toll the
bell," Wilkins says. Wilkins and Bronston got a similar reaction from the Staten Island Medical Society. "We didn't per-

suade one person in that room," Wilkins says. Staten Island was a conservative borough in Nixon's America, and the Fanon Collective didn't exactly blend in. "We were, like, with the Red Book, and Mao Tse Tung and Ho Chi Minh and Huey Newton and Malcolm X on big posters on the wall of our house. It was pretty easy to figure out where we stood."

"We were hated, you know, really hated," Wilkins says. Threatening phone calls came in the middle of the night, and at one point a car was parked outside his apartment all the time. "In the mail I got a picture of myself in a coffin, my head in a coffin," Wilkins says. He never found out who sent it. For a while Wilkins carried a gun, but it just made him even more jittery.

The tide began to turn when Wilkins and Bronston began meeting with the parents of Willowbrook children. Diana McCourt remembers how she got involved. It started on a tour of the Willowbrook grounds. McCourt felt that something about the place wasn't quite right, but she didn't know who to confide in. It was the 1970s, and when McCourt spotted a young man with long hair, she decided he might be the one. His name was Ira Fisher and he was a social worker. Fisher took McCourt aside and said, "I'll talk to you later. There are meetings going on, and I'll bring you to them and tell you about them." Those meetings turned out to be potlucks organized by Wilkins, Bronston, and some sympathetic social workers, who were telling parents about the horrifying conditions behind the locked doors. Soon the parents were not only demanding better treatment for their children but marching in protests. Jane Kurtin, a reporter with the *Staten Island Advance*, investigated the abuses in a series called "What's Wrong with Willowbrook."[18]

It was around this time that the Willowbrook administrators began to panic. The dissenting group of parents was planning a rally for the New Year when Wilkins was called into the office of a supervisor. Jack Hammond, the director of Willowbrook, had ordered the supervisor to fire him. "Dr. Wilkins, you know, you're being terminated," the supervisor said. Wilkins was shocked. He had been told to stop meeting with parents, but he never actually expected to lose his job. Wilkins would later learn that a social worker, Elizabeth Lee, had been fired as well. Wilkins simply told the supervisor, "Oh, okay," and went to empty out his tiny office under the stairs. "He was just doing his job," Wilkins says of the supervisor. "His hand was shaking as he handed me my pencil."

Firing Wilkins was Hammond's first mistake. His second was forgetting to ask Wilkins for his keys. The next day Wilkins called Geraldo Rivera, an attorney-turned-reporter he had met a year or two earlier. Before Wilkins joined the Willow-brook staff, he and the Fanon Collective had worked with the Young Lords, a Puerto Rican civil rights group with roots as a street gang. The Collective had helped the Young Lords set up a screening program for children with lead poisoning. Rivera, a civil rights attorney, had once defended Wilkins after he was arrested. Rivera had left his law practice for a new career as a reporter for a local ABC television affiliate. On an early Jan-uary morning in 1972, Wilkins and Rivera met at a diner on Staten Island and made a plan. They would visit one of the locked wards at Willowbrook with a camera crew.

Rivera and his crew encountered a graphic scene. Naked, emaciated children crouched on the floor of a bare room, the air fetid, the walls smeared with feces. The room was so dark that at first Rivera could scarcely believe what he was seeing. "Welcome to Willowbrook," Wilkins told him.[19] Rivera later compared the experience to what American soldiers must have felt in 1945 when they entered the first concentration camps. "That sound, the mournful wail that the kids were making, is the soundtrack of my nightmares," he said.[20] It took only ten minutes for the crew to film what they needed. Rivera postponed an interview he had scheduled with Hammond and rushed the footage to the studio before anyone could lodge an objection. His first report aired that night.

Rivera's report galvanized the public. Within weeks, the group was meeting with attorneys. The Dick Cavett Show aired a segment on Willowbrook with Wilkins, Bronston, and others as guests.[21] John Lennon raised $1.5 million for Willowbrook in a benefit concert at Madison Square Garden.[22] In March of 1972, the parents of five thousand children filed a class-action lawsuit, *New York ARC v. Rockefeller.*[23]

When I ask Wilkins how so many people could treat the Willowbrook children so poorly for so long, he answers philosophically. "I think they considered them subhuman." He points out that there was a word for children like this in the Middle Ages. "A changeling. A human without a soul." If mentally disabled children can't think or feel the way the rest of us do, they don't demand the same kind of moral response. "That's a concept that I thought was operative at Willowbrook," Wilkins says. "You don't have to think of them as having rights."

I can't disagree with his answer. It is surprisingly easy to see other people as subhuman, even if we rarely put it in those words. I feel myself doing it every time I walk past a homeless person sprawled unconscious on the sidewalk. As a third-year medical student at the Charleston County Hospital, I can remember being assigned a semiconscious elderly patient with the instructions: "Think of her as a plant. You are the gardener. Your job is to keep the plant watered." But this answer explains only so much. The real question is not whether the staff of Willowbrook saw the children as subhuman, but what led them to see them that way.

• • •

The Willowbrook State School opened in 1947 on a 375-acre campus in the Willowbrook section of Staten Island. It was originally planned as a facility for mentally disabled children, but it was used as an army hospital during World War II before the children moved in. Willowbrook was built to house 4,275 residents. By the time Henry Beecher wrote about the hepatitis study in 1966, its population exceeded six thousand. Crowded, dirty, and underfunded, Willowbrook was the largest facility for people with mental disabilities in the country. New York Senator Robert Kennedy visited Willowbrook in 1965 and called it a "snake pit."[24]

If Erving Goffman had ever visited Willowbrook, he would have called it a "total institution." Goffman introduced that phrase in *Asylums*, his pioneering sociological study of institutionalized psychiatric patients.[25] A central organizing feature of modern society, Goffman wrote, is that we tend to sleep, play, and work in different places. We sleep in houses, trailers, and apartments; we play in casinos, gyms, and art studios; we work in offices, hospitals, and police stations. These spaces are not just physically separate. In each one we move among different people and answer to different authorities.

In a total institution, the walls separating these spaces have been dismantled. Every aspect of daily life in a total institution occurs in the same place, under the same authority, in the company of the same people. Examples include psychiatric hospitals, prisons, military units, and boarding schools. In total institutions, the activities of daily life are often rigidly scheduled and enforced by explicit formal rules. These enforced activities are brought together under the umbrella of a single rational plan intended to advance the aims of the institution itself.

Chief among these aims are surveillance and control. The genius of total institutions is how efficiently they allow a relatively small number of staff members to handle a much larger population of inmates, whether those inmates are prisoners, students, or patients. The main job of staff members in total institutions is to see that everyone does what is required of them. This job is made easier under conditions where "one person's infractions stand out in relief against the visible, constantly examined compliance of the others."[26]

A copy of Goffman's *Asylums* was included in the box of books Mike Wilkins loaned to me, as well as a photocopy of Morton Hunt's *New Yorker* article about Pilgrim State Hospital. I can see why Hunt's article made such an impression. Opened in 1931, Pilgrim was not so much a total institution as a total planned community. Pilgrim had its own post office, church, police department, fire department, power plant, commuter rail station, and cemetery. Working there were over thirty-nine hundred staff members, including ninety psychiatrists, seventy-two carpenters, twenty-two barbers, and a shoe repair man. With nearly fourteen thousand psychiatric patients, Pilgrim State Hospital was roughly the same size as Scarsdale, New York.

The grounds of Pilgrim were built according to a standard design used at Willowbrook and other institutions of that period. Hunt describes a scene in Building 1, one of Pilgrim's many H-shaped, two-story buildings. "The men sat immobile, their faces so devoid of expression as to seem featureless. They were of different ages, but were all thoroughly rumpled, useless and wrecked," he writes. The dayroom in one building reminded Hunt of a dungeon, or maybe a debtor's prison. He writes that "the mood conveyed was a total abandonment of hope and slow decay of essential humanity." Hunt could have been describing what Wilkins saw at Willowbrook a decade later.

Total institutions have enabled some of the worst medical research abuses of the modern era. At the Allan Memorial Institute, a psychiatric hospital in Montreal, Dr. Ewen Cameron subjected vulnerable patients to a brutalizing array of experimental interventions, ranging from LSD and repetitive high-voltage electroconvulsive therapy to sodium amytal and months-long induced comas.[27] The University of Pennsylvania dermatologist Albert Kligman did much of his research in Holmesburg Prison. From the 1950s through the 1970s Kligman exposed functionally illiterate, mostly Black inmates to carcinogens, chemical warfare agents, viruses, fungi, and radioisotopes. Many of them suffered severe health problems for the remainder of their lives. Kligman famously described his thoughts on his first visit to Holmesburg: "All I saw before me were acres of skin. It was like a farmer seeing a fertile field for the first time."[28]

It is unlikely that medical researchers go into these institutions with a conscious intention to exploit the inmates. The appeal of total institutions is based on pragmatic concerns. Where else could a researcher find such a population of subjects so compliant and easy to monitor? The subjects live together under one roof. Surveillance is cheap and efficient. Authorities can control the medications, diet, and sleep schedule of each inmate. Every physiological variable can be measured and quantified. It is no wonder that Krugman was tempted by Willowbrook. Not even a university laboratory could offer conditions like this.

Yet the very characteristics that make total institutions so appealing to researchers make them treacherous for subjects. Locked doors and security guards close off the institution from the outside world. Abuses are easy to conceal and difficult for external agencies to monitor. Many total institutions operate under rigid hierarchies that constrain the autonomy of inmates. If inmates are placed under the authority of an institutional officer with absolute power over every aspect of their lives—officers who can reward them, punish them, and determine when (if ever) they will be released from the institution—then they have incentives to please that officer if they ever are asked to sign a consent form.

In total institutions, a bright line separates staff members and inmates. Staff members work shifts and can live normal lives outside the institution, while inmates are usually confined to the institution at all times. The relationship between staff members and inmates is often adversarial. Each side tends to view the other according to hostile stereotypes. Staff members see inmates as secretive, bitter, and duplicitous; inmates see staff members as patronizing, self-righteous, and mean. Staff members accept their place at the top of the status hierarchy and feel as if they deserve it. Inmates tend to feel guilty and inferior.

From a position at the bottom of the status hierarchy, inmates often find their sense of agency slipping away. Institutional norms slowly creep into their unconscious. If someone else is making every decision for you—if your very identity has been stripped away and replaced with that of an "inmate"— then the faculties necessary for self-determination start to seep away as well. It is not just that the authorities regiment and control your daily life, from sleep to meals to recreation. Their control even extends to what Goffman calls the "expressive" aspects of life, those personal choices that express something about your individuality. If, say, the authorities command you to write at least one letter home a week or forbid you from expressing hostility or sullenness, then you will experience the "terror of feeling radically demoted in the age-grading system."[29]

Doctors face the opposite problem. From their perch at the top of the ladder, they are confronted with the temptations of power. Mike Wilkins could see this happening well before he took a job at Willowbrook. Medical training indoctrinates doctors into a class system, he says. "It's mostly on rounds where this class strata comes across. These are the patients; we're the doctors; and there's not an equal relationship. We're not in their class. They're in a separate lower class." By the time medical trainees are in their second year of residency, they have become different people. No longer do they see patients as fellow human beings with equal standing. "They're tarnished in some way," Wilkins says. The doctors have come to think of themselves as the aristocrats, with all the entitlement, privilege, and unshakable sense of superiority conferred by their title.

Wilkins held on to his humanity at Willowbrook, but it wasn't easy. "It was a bad, dirty place where people were suffering on a large scale," he says. A nauseating stench permeated every corner of the institution. Sometimes, when Wilkins was on call, he had to go into buildings that he had never visited before to treat children who had been injured or beaten up. "And it was the same shit, different building," he says. "You know, just people going berserk." In retrospect, Wilkins wonders how many children were having adverse reactions to the drugs they were given. "And some of the time I would be giving them *more* drugs," he says, shaking his head.

Wilkins pauses for a moment. "I didn't know," he says. "You know, you just do a lot of bad things, and you see a lot of bad stuff."

• • •

I am sitting across from Wilkins at a rickety table at the Hard Times Cafe in Minneapolis. It is a cloudy spring day in 2019, and we're here with Niki Gjere, my friend and ally from the Markingson case, who still works at the hospital up the street. My mind is wandering just a little when I hear Wilkins say, "I used to hang out with this crack whore who lived in a tent beneath an underpass." Now I am fully alert. "She wouldn't stay in a shelter," Wilkins says. "She had a tent." The tent sat next to the freeway, yet this woman never hesitated to light up her crack pipe in full view of anyone passing by. Wilkins asked her once if she wasn't afraid of being seen. "Nobody wants to see me, Mike," she said. If everyone averts their eyes, a person might as well be invisible. "That estrangement, I resonate with that," Wilkins says. "I think a lot of people with mental illness bear that burden."

It has been a few months since I first managed to track Wilkins down. Although there wasn't much trace of him on the Internet, I had cold-called a home phone number in Kansas City and got lucky. Wilkins has lived in Kansas City ever since he left Willowbrook in 1974. We planned to meet near his home, but shortly before the date arrived, Wilkins sent me an email saying he needed to cancel. "Yesterday, I had a loving intervention by my wife and all my kids," he wrote. "I have been sad and withdrawn recently and they came up with a plan." Wilkins was starting therapy for post-traumatic stress disorder (PTSD) as well as a day treatment program for his addiction to crack. He said he felt relieved.

Today Wilkins appears healthy and upbeat. He arrived in Minneapolis two days ago to visit his daughter, Erin, who, by coincidence, lives in my neighborhood. Wilkins has finished an intensive five-week course of treatment for PTSD and substance abuse, and by all accounts he is doing well. We've spent the past few days talking about his time at Willowbrook. He brought along several large boxes of papers, books, videocassettes, and photographs, and we've been going through them together in the dining room of my house. Every afternoon he has attended sessions for his addiction with a local twelve-step program.

That trauma can cause lasting psychological damage has been recognized for a long time, but the formal diagnosis of PTSD emerged in the 1970s to describe symptoms sometimes experienced by veterans returning from Vietnam: terrifying flashbacks, disturbing dreams, emotional numbness, unshakable feelings of distrust, a sense of hypervigilance that could explode into violence. Many veterans medicated their symptoms with drugs and alcohol. As a VA employee, Wilkins knew

the symptoms of PTSD well before he was given the diagnosis himself. "Well, you know Vietnam vets are famous for it,"
Wilkins says. "I can spot them a mile away, walking down the
hall, they mostly have a beard—and I, in fact, grew a beard
right as I left New York. I had kept that beard for seventeen
years, and had trouble sleeping, with dreams and these flashbacks, visual and auditory of the scenes in Willowbrook."
What appears in those flashbacks are disturbing images of
children. "Just opening the door, and then seeing them. There
were big metal doors, and they would come at me, you know,"
Wilkins says.

According to the traditional view, PTSD is a psychiatric
disorder that results from trauma and fear. But in an influential 1994 book, *Achilles in Vietnam*, the psychiatrist Jonathan
Shay argued that the trauma experienced by Vietnam veterans resulted not primarily from fear but from being placed in
circumstances where they were commanded to betray widely
held moral standards. Drawing on Homer's epic war poem
The Iliad, Shay compared the experience of Vietnam vets to
that of Achilles, who betrays his sense of what is right when
he follows the commands of his superior, Agamemnon. Such
moral betrayals can cause deep, lasting damage to a person's
character. Shay called this damage "moral injury" and argued
that it was more traumatic than anything else experienced by
combat veterans. "Veterans can usually recover from horror,
fear and grief once they return to civilian life, so long as 'what's
right' has not also been violated," Shay wrote.[30]

What made the war in Vietnam so morally traumatic were
two related forms of violence. First, as a matter of policy,
American military strategy included the deliberate massacre
of civilians, including women and children. Such a policy was
not entirely new, of course. In World War II, the American military had fire-bombed Dresden and dropped atomic bombs on
Hiroshima and Nagasaki. But the American policy in Vietnam

was considered by other nations to be very close to genocide. Second, at least some soldiers took part in unplanned, gratuitous acts of violence against civilians. The massacre at My Lai is a notorious example, but many other veterans came home with stories almost as horrifying. In a guerilla war, where the lines between civilians and combatants can be hard to distinguish, even well-intentioned soldiers could find themselves committing acts that were hard to rationalize when they returned to civilian life.

If a war is widely agreed to be necessary and just, then most veterans can survive the experience psychologically intact. It is much different when the war is barbaric and senseless. According to Shay, the moral injury felt by some veterans comes not from killing the enemy, but from dishonoring them. One veteran had flashbacks of cutting up the corpse of an enemy soldier "just to see what his lungs looked like." Another had intrusive memories every holiday season that centered on a "dead Gook we hung on a tree with a big banner that said, 'Merry Fucking Christmas.'"[31] These soldiers were taught to see the enemy as less than human in order to lessen the trauma of killing, yet paradoxically, this wound up making the trauma even worse. As one veteran told Shay, there is no honor in killing subhuman vermin. Only when a soldier sees the enemy as an honorable adversary can the trauma of war be healed.[32]

Shay emphasized moral betrayals by figures of authority. His paradigm was a military leader who ordered soldiers to carry out actions that are morally condemned by the culture at large, such as killing children or prisoners of war. One patient, a devout Catholic, told Shay the worst experience he had in Vietnam was when he was told to murder seventeen unarmed, nonresisting prisoners. What tormented him was not just that he had willingly followed the order. It was that he had also egged on the other members of his unit, who were reluctant to follow suit. "He calmly carried the certainty that he personally was damned," Shay wrote, "but found it impossible to live with the knowledge that he had led the other marines into mortal sin."[33]

Other scholars see moral injury in terms that are larger and more personal, arguing that injury can result not just from following orders but when any kind of outside pressure forces people to betray their own deeply held moral ideals. In 1984, well before *Achilles in Vietnam*, the philosopher Andrew Jameton developed the concept of "moral distress" to describe the condition of nurses forced to work under morally objectionable circumstances. Nurses may find themselves in dangerously understaffed units, for instance, or participating in what they consider to be futile, painful interventions on dying patients. Moral distress, Jameton wrote, arises "when one knows the right thing to do, but institutional constraints make it nearly impossible to pursue the right course of action."[34]

What kind of psychological injury does whistleblowing cause? The fact that whistleblowers are often condemned for staying true to their moral convictions leaves some of them deeply conflicted. Wilkins can remember how tense and jittery he felt when he was agitating to improve conditions at Willowbrook. "We knew in our heads we were doing something good, but no one else thought it," he says. Instead of feeling proud, he felt guilty and ashamed, even fearful. "You feel like you're going to be punished," he says. "You know, like in *Huckleberry Finn*, where Huck and Jim were riding down the Mississippi, and Huck is saying, 'I know I'm going to go to hell because my preacher says I'm helping this man escape and God wants him to be a slave.'"

Fred Alford has suggested that the wounds of whistleblowers often come from a kind of profound demoralization. Before blowing the whistle, their worldview rested on a solid moral foundation. They lived in a universe where peo-

ple didn't lie without reason, where the authorities followed
the rules, where good works were rewarded and crime didn't
pay. That this foundation could simply collapse never even
occurred to them. When it happens, they are lost. The connection between responsibility and blame has vanished. Their
sense of moral direction is scrambled because all the maps are
gone and the signposts have been changed. How do you find
true north when your compass has no needle?

This kind of foundational collapse is not just crushed idealism. It comes closer to a loss of meaning. Imagine a character
in a Frank Capra movie who finds himself in a film noir. It is
not that the world in *It's a Wonderful Life* is free of disappointment, corruption, or failure. Henry Potter is a villain straight
out of Dickens, and George Bailey nearly throws himself off a
bridge. But it is a world that makes moral sense. The choice
between good and evil is plain. No one is confused about what
constitutes a successful life or a failure. In a film noir, nothing
is what it seems. The characters live in a world of shadows and
confusion and blurred moral lines. Fate is random. Everyone
is alone. Justice is an illusion. Forget it, Jake. It's Chinatown.

Wilkins has thought a lot about moral injury. His own came
mostly from the Willowbrook admissions process. When parents brought a child to Willowbrook, Wilkins says, he stayed
silent about what was in store. He didn't mention the injuries, the infectious diseases, the filth, and the neglect. Nor
did he tell parents about the chance that the child would be
sexually abused. "It was common knowledge that there was
sex going on, and not always consensual, and especially for
a new admission, a nice, well-fed young admission," Wilkins
says. He remembers the medical director joking about it at a
staff meeting. "He says, 'There's cornholing going on, huh?'
And he laughs."

For most children, Wilkins could see no possibility of a good
outcome. The parents had come to Willowbrook because they

couldn't keep their child at home, yet Wilkins knew that any child he admitted was going to be changed drastically, probably for the worse. "You're supposed to be improving things for this kid. And you're not. You're putting them in a bad, bad place for the rest of their life," he says. "This kid is going to be fucked either way. You just decide which is the lesser."

For many whistleblowers, the act of blowing the whistle triggers a long slide into despair. But for Wilkins, it felt like redemption. He had already been fired. Blowing the whistle was a way to turn that firing to his advantage. "That was the liberating, the salvaging thing about what we were doing. We had a plan; we were working the plan; and then it actually worked, which was unlikely, but it worked," Wilkins says. That success sets him apart from many other whistleblowers. Wilkins still lives in a moral universe with sense and meaning. He went into Willowbrook as an idealist and came out the same way. "The arc of justice, it's there. It's real," he tells me. "I've got to believe in it; I don't think I can stop believing in it."

Wilkins is proud of what he accomplished at Willowbrook, but he resists my efforts to characterize him as courageous. "I was really dedicated to the struggle, but I'm the world's biggest chicken," he says. "I wouldn't be in a physical fight with anybody. I wouldn't. I'd be afraid. I mean, I'd run from it." He credits his success to the solidarity of his friends and allies in the Fanon Collective. At Willowbrook Wilkins was accompanied by Bill Bronston, a slightly older physician with expertise in mental retardation. Wilkins says, "I would have left that place in a week if I was by myself."

• • •

Bill Bronston is not a whistleblower. He made that clear to me on the phone, and now that I am at his house outside Sacramento, he is making it clear again. "I am a warrior," he says. "A ferocious, organized warrior. I am doing something every minute, all the time, to advance justice." Bronston is showing me around his house, every room of which is filled with original art and sculpture. His thinning silver hair is swept back from his forehead, and over a gray turtleneck he wears a black bead necklace. Ebullient and self-assured, Bronston fills up the room. It is easy to imagine him behind a podium or leading a crowd of protesters. If he were not so warm and gracious, I might feel a little intimidated.

I've driven out to Bronston's house from San Francisco, where my wife, Ina, and I have stopped for a few days on our way to New Zealand. I had hoped to soak up a little gonzo mojo at the Seal Rock Inn, the hotel where Hunter S. Thompson wrote *Fear and Loathing on the Campaign Trail '72*. But the vibe there has been eerily quiet. It is early March of 2020, and the coronavirus is just starting to appear in the news. Each morning we have linguica sausage and scrambled eggs in a near-empty hotel restaurant. A white lawn jockey with an amputated finger stands sentinel at the entrance. From the window we can see the *Diamond Princess* and its hostage crew of COVID-infected passengers hovering off the coast, unable to dock. After breakfast I usually work at the desk in our room, a brown and beige number with wood paneling, industrial green carpet, and a fake fireplace. If you squint, you can imagine it is still 1972.

It's even easier when you hear Bronston hold forth. "Every struggle is the same," he tells me. "Every struggle has its community, has its righteousness, has its compelling heartful purpose, and when you come to people they will leave the comfort and the routine of their lives and help." If Bronston sounds like a man of grand vision, he comes by it honestly. He grew up in a Russian-Jewish household in Hollywood. His father, Samuel Bronston, was a movie producer known for epic films with spectacular sets, such as *King of Kings*, *John Paul Jones*, and *El Cid*, starring Charlton Heston as the legendary Castilian warrior. Bronston's great-uncle was Lev Bronstein, better known as Leon Trotsky. Bronston says he doesn't like to trade on the family connection, but Trotsky's influence is not hard to detect. "It is a very sentimental and moral presence in my life," he says. "I really embrace the need for a socialist revolution."

Like Wilkins, Bronston despised medical school from day one. He chafed at the rigid hierarchies and authoritarian ethos. "I was just thunderstruck at the cultural barrenness of the everyday studies," he says. "There was no talk about the people-ness of who it was that we were serving, or the whole notion of service as opposed to being a high-level mechanic, a plumber." Bronston channeled his anger into the kind of activism that has characterized his entire career. As a student he rallied medical and nursing students across the country to press for curricular change. Later, as a psychiatric resident at the Menninger Clinic in Topeka, Kansas, Bronston was fired after helping reactivate a dormant union of poorly paid psychiatric aides and organizing an action that led to a takeover of several hospital wards. In the 1990s, Bronston fought successfully to get a heart-lung transplant for Sandra Jensen, a thirty-five-year-old woman with Down syndrome.[35] Even now, in his eighties, Bronston is deeply involved in the movement for universal health care. He is still frustrated with his inability to get other doctors on board. "They're chicken shits," he says. "All that privilege and all that status is groundless if they don't have a warrior's soul."

When Bronston started work at Willowbrook, he was appalled by what he saw. "It was truly an American concentration camp," he says. "There weren't more than two workers on a ward with fifteen of the most fucked-up people you can imagine. I mean, people that were just soaked and drowned in tranquilizers." Bronston had worked with mentally disabled children with Richard Koch at the University of South-

ern California. He knew what was possible for such children
and he saw how badly Willowbrook was failing them. "There
were about forty doctors. They were all corrupt. They were all
incompetent. They hated the work. They didn't want to touch
anybody in there."

Yet Bronston is quick to distinguish his reaction to Willowbrook from that of Wilkins. "Mike doesn't look for trouble,"
Bronston says. "He's just a sweetheart. He's just a good guy, a
totally good guy." Bronston sees whistleblowers like Wilkins
as moral innocents, decent people who are hurt when they see
cruelty or injustice. They feel morally compelled to stop the
injustice, but they don't think about dismantling the system
that is propping it up. That's what Bronston wanted to do at
Willowbrook. Genuine reform requires leaders who understand the systemic structures that sustain injustice and have
the tools to bring them crashing down. Bronston has always
aspired to that role—not a whistleblower, but a revolutionary.

This view is evident in the way Bronston recalls the Willowbrook struggle. When Wilkins tells the story of Willowbrook, his tone is pensive and haunted. He remembers small
moments and particular children. Bronston, in contrast, is
passionate. His face lights up when he speaks. He narrates
the struggle in language that is grand and heroic, like El Cid
remembering the conquest of Valencia. "When you're working with tinder and light one match, you don't have to do a lot
to get people to feel themselves and to feel the righteousness
of their care for their own," he says. "These parents were profoundly depressed and guilty and sorrowful and felt powerless, and when that was neutralized, it was replaced with rage
and courage and purpose."

When I hear Bronston remember the struggle, I can easily
imagine him playing the hero's part in one of his father's epics.
It is a rare man who can talk about a "warrior's soul" without
irony. Bronston speaks the language of honor and glory like it

is his native tongue. If he sounds immodest, no one should be surprised. A notable aspect of the honor ethic is how it fuses moral principles with personal ambition. The political philosopher Sharon Krause cites the example of Martin Luther King Jr, whose humble demeanor could sometimes mask his sense of historical importance. In the ethic of honor, there is no contradiction between the pursuit of glory and the righteous aims of the struggle.[36] Ralph Abernathy called King the "peaceful warrior," and King embraced the label. "We did not hesitate to call ourselves an army," King said. "But it was a special army, with no supplies but its sincerity, no uniform but its determination, no arsenal except its faith, no currency but its conscience."[37]

Like Wilkins, Bronston was wounded by the struggle. "I just carry this terrible sadness all the time. I have this ocean of tears and sadness in me," he says. "That's part of the flotation device for my activism." Yet Bronston doesn't carry the burden of guilt and moral injury that Wilkins does. "That's sort of how I'm different from Michael. I mean, I knew that there was nothing that I could do on an individual basis anywhere." Bronston speaks of his wounds as if they are the inevitable result of revolutionary activism. You follow your conscience, yet you are rejected and reviled. Those kinds of wounds stay with you even if you succeed. "What happens is that you are profoundly moved by how accidental and how it could have gone any other way," he says. "You didn't have to win. The fact that you won was at some level a total accident."

As different as Wilkins and Bronston are, they share a moral sensibility that allowed them to see Willowbrook for what it was. They didn't see it as a research laboratory, as Krugman did. They didn't see the children as subhuman creatures to be treated like farm animals. They saw fellow human beings in need of help. That view may seem natural to anyone who has watched *Willowbrook: The Last Great Disgrace*, yet it put them at odds with every other physician at Willowbrook. What I wanted from Bronston was an explanation—not so much for why he and Wilkins saw the reality of Willowbrook, but rather, why no one else did.

For Bronston, the explanation begins with the architecture. "The buildings tell the story," he says. When you set foot into a new place for the first time, with no firm sense of how to behave, you look around for cues. And the first cues come from the very structure of the institution—how it is built, the way it is organized, what people are doing. You simply assume there is a good reason things are arranged as they are, whether the institution is a nursing home, a prison, or a psychiatric ward. "The place speaks to the legitimacy of the model and to the role and the status of the people in the model more loudly than anything else imaginable," Bronston says. "Medically secured, medically managed, doctor-validated. If it's going that way, it's because it's okay. Because if it wasn't okay, it wouldn't be going that way."

It rarely occurs to anyone to object, especially not students or residents. "You go in there and you say, 'Who am I to raise a question?' The question of even raising the question is not an option. You go in there humbly to kind of get it, to just kind of get with the program. You get with the program because that's what you're being hired to do," Bronston says. It's not necessarily that you are so hard-hearted that you feel nothing when you see human suffering. It's just that the feeling goes no further. "Your heart is broken. And you go back to class and that's the end of it. And it is what it is, and it stays there, and nobody says, 'How is this possible? How is this possible for people to be treated like this? How is it possible for professionals to be complicit in this kind of behavior?'"

Bronston understands how it is possible, at least for the physicians at Willowbrook. "They were old. They needed the job. It was not hard work. They could come and go as they wished. They were collaborators, just like Nazi collaborators, you know. I mean, you get paid and you're in the paradigm. They accepted the paradigm. You walk into the place, and everything says, 'This is okay, because the problem of the people there is mental retardation.' So you walk in there, and you see what you are defined to see as mental retardation—hopeless, helpless, unfixable, you know, broken, trashed people—and then you're there to help." So you help a little, and then a little more, and pretty soon you have a routine. Without quite realizing it, you've become part of the machine. "You think you're helping," Bronston says, "but all you're doing is complicitly legitimizing this abuse, this crime against humanity."

As I listen to Bronston, I wonder whether one reason he and Wilkins could see what was invisible to other doctors is that they both hated medical school. Part of what makes medical training so unnerving is how frequently you are thrust into new settings in which you don't really know how to behave. Nothing in your previous life has prepared you to euthanize a dog in the physiology laboratory, or help deliver a round of electroconvulsive therapy on a nonconsenting patient, or attempt an episiotomy on a sixteen-year-old girl without anesthesia. Is this normal? Are we supposed to be doing this? Maybe, but maybe not. It's hard to tell. Your gut reaction is often a combination of anxiety, revulsion, and social discomfort. Most people learn to suppress that reaction. A rare few learn from it.

. . .

Wilkins and I are finishing up our walk in Kansas City. There is still a morning chill in the air as we walk past Union Cemetery. Wilkins is telling me about his departure from Staten Island in 1972. "I had PTSD and didn't know it. I just knew what I couldn't stand to be around. And anything that had to do with Willowbrook was one of those things. And even the

Collective. I left it with very little notice of the reason why. I got married to a woman who worked at the Westchester County organization for mentally retarded children. That lasted six months," he says. Wilkins came back to Kansas City and threw himself into his internal medicine residency. Over time he came to understand himself better. He has been married to Jody for forty years and they have five children now, all grown. "I am not a big picture guy," he says. "I'm a one patient at a time guy. That's my role. I know that. I know that I love doing that," he says.

As we walk, I ask Wilkins about a story he mentioned earlier. From a very early age, his mother had absolutely insisted that he was a good and kind person. Because of her unwavering belief, Wilkins says, he gradually became that person. "It's true," he tells me. It started when Wilkins helped a younger girl who had fallen and hurt herself. "Everyone else just walked on, but I stayed and helped her," he says. Afterward, the girl's mother called up Mike's mother and told her the story. "My mom jumped on that as proof positive that I was a saint. And she really did believe that," he says. "That was her position." Wilkins says he has tried to do the same thing with his own children.

In a small way, this story illustrates how honor often works. By virtue of what you are told about yourself, you develop a story about the kind of person you are. You develop expectations of yourself based at least partly on what others see in you. If you meet those expectations, you feel proud, and if you fail, you feel ashamed. Your story isn't written in stone, of course, and it doesn't usually come solely from one person. But sometimes it takes only one person to put the story in your head. You are told you are kind, and you become kind. You are admired for your courage, and you become courageous. You are given a role, and eventually you inhabit the role so thoroughly that the role and the actor are one.

Wilkins understands that his role is not that of a revolutionary. His role is that of a doctor who knows his patients and hears their stories and bears witness to their suffering. "I'm going to be out there on the street. I'm going to be out there with the thieves and beggars and addicts," he says. Not many of his medical colleagues are aware of what he did at Willowbrook. He is not the sort of person who would tell a story in which he has done the honorable thing. "I don't talk about it. I don't bring it up, because it gets tiresome talking about it," he says. "Why should I? I mean, life goes on." He pauses. "It's like if you have a hit song, you don't want to keep singing it."

CHAPTER 4

The Hutch

No matter how hard you try, it's hard to put a hopeful spin on the story of John Pesando's struggle against the Fred Hutchinson Cancer Research Center. There is no silver lining, no triumph over long odds, no hard-earned lesson about the unbreakable human spirit. His is a bleak, demoralizing story of defeat. Pesando is the first to insist on telling it this way. For years he attempted to expose abuses of cancer patients at the Hutch, where he worked as a young researcher and clinician. No one would take his concerns seriously—not the authorities at the Hutch, nor those at regulatory agencies, nor those in the state or federal government. For many years, not even journalists would respond. When Pesando finally found reporters at the *Seattle Times* who would listen, their reporting changed nothing. Neither did litigation. "It was astounding that nobody gave a damn," Pesando tells me. "So that was probably one of the most shocking things, that nobody really gave a shit. And I wasn't prepared for that."

Pesando and I are sitting 6 feet apart on a park bench in

the Capitol Hill neighborhood of Seattle. It is a chilly September afternoon, but the park is lush and verdant, with a clear view of Lake Union in the distance. Pesando is a slender man with a gray, neatly clipped mustache. He grew up in Ontario, and his accent still contains slight Canadian undertones. (He pronounces "again" as "a gain.") Something about his manner suggests understated competence and efficiency, like a helpful curator at the Library of Congress or maybe an experienced forester at a national park. He doesn't reveal much about himself. Occasionally he will make a dark, cynical joke, and then his face breaks out into a boyish grin, and he looks downward a little shyly as he laughs. He is wearing a Patagonia jacket and a flat cap of the type I usually associate with London taxi drivers.

Pesando was thirty-six years old in 1982 when he took up a position at the Hutch. His career up to that point had been a steady climb upward to the highest levels of academic medicine: a magna cum laude undergraduate degree from Harvard, an MD and PhD from the Albert Einstein College of Medicine, a residency at the University of Pennsylvania, an assistant professorship at Harvard and the Dana Farber Cancer Institute in Boston. All that changed when Pesando moved to the Hutch and was asked to serve on the IRB. There he learned about an ongoing cancer study of bone marrow transplantation called Protocol 126. Like other members of the IRB, Pesando was alarmed by the study. Unlike the others, he couldn't forget about it. He tried to blow the whistle on the study for nearly two decades.

"I was naive," Pesando says. "I was like an eighteen-year-old going off to fight a war somewhere." His moral innocence will become a running theme in our conversations. As Pesando tells it, his attitude toward institutions and figures of authority back then was one of idealism and misplaced trust. He assumed the best of other people and believed they would do the right thing. "I thought the world would be concerned and take corrective action if I went out on a limb," Pesando says. He was mistaken. He lost his job and his research career, while one of the men he accused of misconduct went on to win a Nobel Prize. He says, "I wish I had been more cynical."

Our meeting on this Seattle park bench has been a long time coming. Although I met Pesando a few years ago, we have not yet had an extended conversation about his experience as a whistleblower. Our first setback was the coronavirus. The pandemic had arrived in March 2020, and months passed before I felt as if a road trip to Seattle could be accomplished safely. But when Ina, my wife, and I finally left Minneapolis, wildfires were blazing out of control in the West. Almost as soon as we hit the road, warnings from our friends in the Pacific Northwest began to arrive: "The sun has vanished. You can't venture outside. Your throat will burn. It feels like something from the Book of Revelation. Stay away."

And so we did. All through Montana and Wyoming we drove, waiting for the smoke in Seattle to clear. We picked our daily destination largely by air quality forecasts and COVID infection rates. At daybreak we would check the Purple Air and Accuweather websites for a spot with breathable air, and then we would search on Kayak and Airbnb to find a new place to stay: Bozeman, Cody, Pinedale, Yellowstone, Helena. Every time I emailed Pesando, hoping for an improved weather forecast, his replies were dark and pessimistic. It was a week of foreboding news and exhaustive Internet searches, followed by long drives through vast western landscapes. There was something almost biblical about the journey: wandering in the wilderness, our travels driven by pestilence and plague.

What is unusual about Pesando's story is not that he failed to stop an objectionable study or get any justice for the victims. That result is depressingly common. It is that he learned about the study through his service on the Institutional

Review Board. These oversight bodies were set up in the wake of the Tuskegee study. IRB members have a broad view of potentially unethical research. Often they get a rare glimpse into the darkest, most dangerous corners of a research institution. If they see subjects in danger of harm or exploitation, it is their duty to protect them. It was Pesando's misfortune to find himself on an IRB that was either unwilling or unable to do that. At first he resisted internally; eventually, he went public. Perhaps there are other research scandals that were exposed by an IRB member, but I haven't been able to find them.

As Pesando and I talk together on the park bench, our conversation is interrupted by an unusual noise. A crowd of two dozen people or so have gathered nearby, and one of them is blowing a ceremonial horn. "Rosh Hashanah," Pesando says, and now the scene makes sense. It is the Jewish New Year, and the coronavirus has driven the ceremony outdoors. The ram's horn, or shofar, is what Joshua and the Israelites blew to bring down the walls of Jericho. Joshua was following a command from God. I wonder: What would Joshua have done if he had blown his shofar and the walls of Jericho had simply stood firm, refusing to collapse?

• • •

The scandal of Protocol 126 was broken on March 11, 2001, by Duff Wilson and David Heath, two investigative reporters for the *Seattle Times*. Their series was called "Uninformed Consent," and the story they told was grim.[1] For twelve years, a team of researchers at the Hutch had attempted a type of experimental bone marrow transplantation on patients with leukemia and lymphoma. Many of the patients would have had a good chance of cure with standard, nonexperimental treatment—in some cases, as high as 60 percent. Yet by the time Protocol 126 ended, eighty-four of the eighty-five subjects were dead.[2] At least twenty patients had died of graft failure—a disastrous consequence that ordinarily occurs in less than 1 percent of bone marrow transplantation recipients.

According to the *Seattle Times,* the struggle over Protocol 126 began on January 20, 1981, when three cancer researchers at the Hutch submitted the study for ethical approval by the Hutch's Institutional Review Board.[3] (At the time, it was called the Human Subjects Review Committee.) Protocol 126 was intended to treat a problem called graft-versus-host disease (GVHD), a problem unique to the transplantation of bone marrow. In conventional transplants, such as kidney or heart transplants, the major barrier is that the recipient's body will recognize the donor's organ as foreign and reject it. But bone marrow transplantation also carries a risk of the reverse: that the donated bone marrow will recognize the recipient's body as foreign and attack it. In the early 1980s, as many as half of the recipients of transplants from tissue-matched sibling donors suffered GVHD. Often the symptoms were mild, such as a skin rash, but in 5 to 10 percent of patients, the condition could be fatal.[4]

The researchers were Paul Martin, a young oncologist; John Hansen, his mentor; and Donnall Thomas, a legendary figure at the Hutch who had been involved in the very first bone marrow transplant decades earlier. They believed that GVHD was enabled by T cells in the donor marrow. If those T cells were depleted before the donor marrow was transplanted, the researchers believed, the risk of GVHD could be diminished. They planned to kill the T cells with monoclonal antibodies—antibodies manufactured by cloning a unique white blood cell. Afterward they would transplant the T cell–depleted bone marrow in the usual way. By early 1981, the researchers were ready to test this theory in humans. All they needed was a green light from the IRB.

The meeting of January 20, 1981 would mark the start of an astonishing twelve-year exchange between the IRB and the

Protocol 126 researchers. It didn't begin with a green light. In fact, the light was flashing red. So alarming were the flaws in Protocol 126 that the IRB initially refused to let the study proceed. Yet not only did the IRB reverse its decision within three months and approve Protocol 126, but it would also continue to approve modified versions of the study for twelve more years, even as the death count soared.

In its very first review, the IRB flagged the critical problem with Protocol 126: graft failure. The IRB worried that removing T cells from the donor marrow would increase the risk that the recipient's body would fail to accept the transplanted bone marrow. If that happened, the subject would probably die. To make matters worse, the researchers had targeted a subject population at very low risk of GVHD in the first place. To the IRB, it did not appear that the researchers had done enough research on animals to proceed to human studies. "The jump from mouse to man is too great," one IRB member said.[5]

Under ordinary circumstances, a rejection by the IRB would have been enough to stop the study in its tracks. At the very least it would prompt significant changes. But these researchers were not deterred. Three months later, they resubmitted Protocol 126 to the IRB with only minor revisions. This time the IRB said yes. Exactly why the IRB changed its mind is unclear. A similar kind of back-and-forth would repeat itself for over a decade. With each transplant failure or rejection would come another tweak to the experiment; with each new worry expressed by the IRB would come another round of negotiations. In the end, however, Protocol 126 was an utter failure. Nearly everyone enrolled in the study would die. According to the *Seattle Times*, at least twenty of the subjects died from causes attributable to the study.[6]

Did the subjects in Protocol 126 really understand the risks they were taking? That question emerged more than once in the exchanges between the researchers and the IRB, especially when the subjects began to die. "The informed consent should at the very least indicate that some unexpected adverse effects have occurred," one IRB member wrote in 1983, understating the issue considerably.[7] Several members of the IRB found the consent forms misleading. They pressed the researchers to state explicitly that if the first bone marrow graft failed, it was extremely unlikely that a second attempt would succeed.

Dan Johnson, one of the attorneys who became involved in litigation against the Hutch, is brutal in his assessment of the study. "There was a bait and switch," Johnson tells me. Most of the research subjects represented by Johnson's firm had come to the Hutch from other parts of the country. "These are people in their middle age who get leukemia and whose chances at the time of survival were, you know, 30, 40, 50, 60 up to 85 percent with the standard treatment depending on the particulars of their case," he says. The patients had chosen the Hutch over other leading cancer centers, often after visiting or talking to representatives of the Hutch on the phone. "At no time during that process were they told that they would get anything but the standard transplant," Johnson says.

After the bait came the switch. Once patients had decided on the Hutch, these patients booked their flights and hotel rooms and brought their families to Seattle. But according to Johnson, it was only after the patients had checked into the hospital and had a Hickman catheter surgically placed that they were asked to sign up for Protocol 126. "I mean, it's the day the treatment begins when they sit down with the doctor and discuss this protocol," Johnson says. "To me that's pretty outrageous, because that's not a person or a family that's in a position to really weigh options. You know, they've already made their choices."

Paul Martin, the only living member of the Protocol 126 research team, is still on the faculty of the Hutch. When I asked Martin by phone if he had any regrets about how the study proceeded, he said no. "I think, if anything, that we were convinced that we could make it work," he said. "I'm seventy-two now, and so I know a heck of a lot more than I did, just from experience, but you know, the only way you can learn what works and what doesn't work is by trying it." He conceded that they may have persevered a little longer than they should have, but he pointed out that this is a retrospective judgment. "You know, it's a human tendency to keep trying," he said.

• • •

John Pesando remembers the exact moment when he was summoned to join the IRB. It was a sunny August day, and he was working in his office in Eklind Hall. A faint smell of urine hung in the air, courtesy of a mouse laboratory located nearby. John Mills, an administrator, brought the message. The Hutch had just reconstituted its IRB and combined it with a similar body at Swedish Medical Center, in Seattle. The director of the Hutch wanted Pesando to join.

Pesando was not exactly thrilled to get this invitation. The work of an IRB is demanding if you take it seriously. Meetings typically take place once a month, and the members must usually read hundreds of pages of dense scientific protocols. There is no status or prestige attached to IRB membership; in many institutions, IRBs are resented if not despised. Pesando politely declined. But Mills made it clear that the invitation was an order, not a request. "I did not want to serve on the IRB," Pesando says. "I was forced to serve."

When Pesando joined the reconstituted IRB in September 1983, Protocol 126 was several months into its most lethal phase. At the time, Pesando had no way of knowing that. Nor did he know about the grave concerns of the previous IRB. What concerned him about Protocol 126 was the absence of basic information. The researchers had not told the IRB what monoclonal antibodies they were using. Pesando found this oversight disturbing. "Basically, every monoclonal antibody is a drug unto itself," Pesando says. "And yet the protocol was approved for generic use of unspecified antibodies to treat bone marrow." He compares the IRB's decision to issuing a blank check. It seemed like a very bad idea.

The new IRB had another concern. There was a rumor at the Hutch about possible financial impropriety. It was said that the three researchers on Protocol 126—Paul Martin, John Hansen, and Donnall Thomas—owned large amounts of stock in Genetic Systems Corporation, the company that licensed the monoclonal antibodies they were using. If this were true, it might constitute a financial incentive for the researchers to push the study forward. To clarify the matter, Henry Kaplan, the chair of the IRB, wrote to Don Thomas. Among his questions was whether "checks and balances" were in place to manage potential financial conflicts of interest.

Thomas was not just another researcher on Protocol 126. He was a pioneer in bone marrow transplantation and the clinical director of the Hutch. Thomas did not welcome Kaplan's questions. "There are no such conflicts," he wrote back. "I think Committee members have not only an obligation to review the ethical aspects of this work, but also an obligation to assist us and not impede our research."[8] Even more ominous, according to Pesando, was the informal feedback the IRB got. At the next meeting, he says, one of the members who was friendly with Thomas told the committee, "Dr. Thomas was pissed." Apparently, Thomas was even angrier than his letter suggested. "There was a hush at the meeting at that point," Pesando says. "There was palpable fear in the meeting when that was announced. Dr. Thomas was like Donald Trump. I mean, he controlled everything. He had a fearsome reputation. You didn't oppose the man."

Pesando says it was the intimidating presence of Thomas that cowed faculty members into remaining silent. "He was all-powerful, basically. Part of it was his reputation as the godfather of bone marrow transplant," Pesando says. "People were afraid of him. Because when you didn't do what he wanted you to do, he took reprisals." Thomas had been the first director of medical oncology when the Hutch opened its doors in 1975. Pesando alternately refers to him as "the 800-pound gorilla," "the cock of the roost," "the Jolly Green Giant," and "the supreme dictator." Curious as to why exactly Thomas was so intimidating, I asked Pesando whether he was especially loud. "No, he was a very soft-spoken man," Pesando replied. "He sort of looked like Santa Claus."

Pesando had moved from Dana Farber to the Hutch in 1982 because of its reputation as a major center for leukemias and lymphomas. But he found the culture of the Hutch chilly and balkanized. "I'm the new kid on the block, and I took a lot of my colleagues, clinical and basic science, out to lunch and so forth, to find what they were doing, what kind of people they were," he says. But there was almost no reciprocity, he says. "It was really spooky how cold the environment was, how unsupportive it was," Pesando says. "I mean, I felt very isolated. You're in the lab, you know, you're spending long hours—eighty-hour weeks were not uncommon—and you're almost like a monk."

A few months after starting on the IRB, Pesando started working on the clinical service for the first time, taking care of cancer patients on the transplantation ward at Swedish Hospital. One of his first patients was Jackie Couch, a thirty-one-year-old lawyer from New Jersey who kept a picture of her young daughter by her bedside. The nurses liked her and so did Pesando. Couch had been treated with chemotherapy for acute myelogenous leukemia (AML) back home and had achieved a complete remission. But most such patients eventually have a recurrence, so Couch had come to the Hutch for a bone marrow transplant. According to her physician, it would offer a 50 percent chance of cure.

When Couch arrived in September, however, she was recruited into Protocol 126. By the time Pesando began taking care of Couch in January 1984, the study had left her in miserable shape. "The medical problem list was just absolutely horrific," Pesando says. Her first bone marrow transplant had failed, and after another grueling course of chemotherapy, Couch had been given a second transplant. Her condition had deteriorated rapidly. Her kidneys and liver had failed, and she had developed ascites as well as a potentially fatal fungal infection. When Pesando took over her care, Couch was on dialysis and getting platelet infusions and intravenous antibiotics. She made it through that crisis, but her improvement was short-lived. After a few months it was clear that the second transplant had failed as well. She died on April 22, 1984.

Jackie Couch was not the only one of Pesando's patients in Protocol 126 to die. Ruth Fisher was a thirty-eight-year-old computer programmer from California with a diagnosis of chronic myelogenous leukemia (CML). Unlike Jackie Couch, Fisher looked relatively healthy when Pesando took over her care. Her first bone marrow transplant in December had failed to engraft, however, and according to Protocol 126, this meant a second transplant. Pesando had seen how badly Jackie Couch had deteriorated after her second transplant, so he went to Rainer Storb, a senior physician, for advice. "I'm concerned because my other patient did so poorly," Pesando said. He says Storb told him, "Don't worry about it. They all die. The grafts always fail in this context." (Storb says he does not recall this conversation).

Pesando was horrified. "And I'm looking at him, and I said, 'You know, this is not what the consent form says. Neither the one I'm reading to her or the one she signed the first time,'" he says. A second transplant was a death sentence. Yet according to Pesando, the consent form made it sound like taking aspirin for a headache. "It's okay to do things to people with their consent, but you tell them to the best of your knowledge what the risks are, what the benefits are," Pesando says. "You don't conceal information in order to sell them something, or to get their permission." Fisher was given a second transplant in mid-January, and eleven days later she was dead. The death hit Pesando very hard. "I got very close to these ladies," he says. "They were charming people."

Unlike many other physicians at the Hutch, Pesando could see Protocol 126 from the air as well as from the ground. As an IRB member, he reviewed the study as an abstract project: the numbers, the statistics, and the scientific data. As a clinician on the Swedish hospital ward, he saw up close what the research subjects were experiencing. Both views disturbed him. Later he learned that Jackie Couch and Ruth Fisher were not the only two deaths in the study. "Turns out there were already five others out there who had similar problems," Pesando says. "I wasn't aware of them. The IRB wasn't aware of them. They weren't reporting to us in a timely fashion. They weren't reporting to us at all."

In fact, the researchers had enrolled at least one subject in Protocol 126 before the IRB had even approved it. David Yingling, a forty-five-year-old insurance agent from Indiana, had come to the Hutch for treatment of acute myelogenous leukemia. His brother donated bone marrow, but the Hutch lost most of it in a laboratory error. Yingling was enrolled in Protocol 126, and what was left of the donor marrow was depleted of T cells. The graft failed, and Yingling died within two months.[9]

Burdened by a sense of responsibility, Pesando decided to bring up his concerns at the next weekly staff meeting, which was led by Don Thomas. "I made a point of saying, 'Sir, we have a problem with Protocol 126. I've had two patients who died on this protocol,'" Pesando says. "And I went into all the technical details of what had happened." When Pesando finished his brief presentation, Thomas just looked at him and said, "Who the hell are you to question what we do around here?" The room fell silent. No other staff member said anything. After a minute or two the discussion moved on to other subjects.

"I mean, that was a shocker," Pesando says. What stunned him more than the put-down by Thomas was the fact that no one in the room spoke up. Pesando had just explained that two subjects in Protocol 126 had died unnecessarily and why he believed that others were going to meet the same fate. Yet once Thomas made it clear where he stood, not a single person was willing to question him. "There was no gathering of equals, no Knights of the Round Table," Pesando says. "The guy with the white beard sat at the end of the table, and everybody else, if they stepped out of line in his opinion, was publicly eviscerated." After that meeting, Pesando could feel the distance between him and the other staff members growing. "I felt like an outsider very quickly," he says.

After his traumatic experience with Couch and Fisher, Pesando could not bear the thought of more subjects being enrolled in Protocol 126. Yet on the transplantation ward, he was still required to give patients the option of enrolling. So Pesando began a covert operation to keep his patients out of the study, telling them that Protocol 126 was a very bad idea. He says he was fairly blunt. "I would say most of the people on this protocol have had graft failure or died with recurrent leukemia," he says, even though this fact wasn't mentioned on the consent form. "The consent form made it sound benign." Afterward, Pesando covered his tracks, because he knew that his superiors would disapprove. "So, my official notes didn't say all the cautionary notes that I told them in person," he says. "Because as I say: Big Brother was watching me."

Pesando's blunt assessment was often enough to deter patients from Protocol 126, but he remembers one patient that he could not talk out of signing up, no matter how hard he tried. He shakes his head as he remembers the conversation. "I remember the explanation she gave me was, 'If it's good enough for the Hutch, it's good enough for me.' I gave her the spiel about 100 percent mortality, but God, she was not to be talked out of it," Pesando says. "She died, of course."

The IRB continued to raise questions about Protocol 126. But in the end, those questions made little difference. The chair, Henry Kaplan, lost his appetite for the fight, according to Pesando. "By the end of that first year, he shut down," Pesando says. "He ceased to have any emotional involvement in the issues put forward." Kaplan would admit much later that he simply trusted that the researchers knew what they were doing. "While I was uneasy about it, I felt these guys were the experts at it," he said. (Kaplan declined my invitation for an interview.) Pesando says he came away from IRB meetings upset and demoralized.

Pesando's own research began to falter. His main federal research grant (his R01, in American medical jargon) was not renewed, and his efforts to get other grants failed. In the world of modern academic medicine, where researchers are expected above all else to be fundraisers, the failure to obtain research dollars is a virtual death knell. Young researchers in need of funding must spend more and more time writing grants rather than doing research; yet time spent away from research makes it hard for them to demonstrate that they are worth an investment. It is easy for a promising research career to spiral downward.

Pesando came to the Hutch with the understanding that he was on the cusp of getting a permanent appointment. But his promotion to that appointment kept getting pushed back. "It just never happened," Pesando says. In February of 1987,

Thomas summoned Pesando to his office and told him that his time at the Hutch was finished. The dismissal essentially ended Pesando's medical research career. He was still in his early forties. Pesando found a consulting position at a biotechnology company in Seattle, but after a short time there, he moved on to a job with the Social Security Administration reviewing disability claims. He has spent the rest of his career there.

Pesando shakes his head when he remembers how Thomas fired him. "You're not a team player," Thomas said. Being a team player apparently meant following orders. When I asked Pesando if the criticism stung, he said no, absolutely not. "Because I wasn't a team player, right? The team is committing Nazi war crimes. Do I want to be a team player? No."

· · ·

One of the great mysteries of crime and sin is how organizations composed of ordinary people can produce behavior that, from the outside, looks unthinkable. Even insiders often struggle afterward to explain why they did what they did. Moral philosophers typically try to understand wrongdoing by looking at individual character and personal choice. A better question would be how organizations create social worlds in which disastrous moral choices seem normal and sensible.

In the early 1980s, the sociologist Robert Jackall conducted fieldwork with managers in several large corporations with the aim of understanding how corporations shape the moral consciousness of their employees. He found the answer in the nature of bureaucracy: that peculiarly modern way of organizing human activity that emerged in the nineteenth century and is now so pervasive that it is almost invisible. Of course, corporate bureaucracies are different from those of hospitals and research institutions, just as they are different from military units, prisons, and public schools. But the influence of the

bureaucratic form today extends to virtually every large organization. As I listened to Pesando talk about his years at the
Hutch, I was struck by the resonance between his descriptions
and the bureaucratic world that Jackall describes in his 1988
book, *Moral Mazes*.[10]

According to standard accounts, bureaucracies are complex organizations composed of trained professionals performing administrative tasks. They are characterized by their
impersonality, their rigid division of labor, and their reliance
on written records and procedures. Rank and hierarchy are
extremely important in bureaucracies; higher-ranking officials supervise subordinates through a prescribed chain of
command. This is a key feature of bureaucracies. As long as
bureaucrats act within prescribed policies and procedures,
they can expect to be insulated from responsibility for the
consequences of their actions.

Bureaucracy shapes consciousness in several different
ways, Jackall explains. It gives people a socially approved,
purpose-driven schedule in which their work is standardized
and made routine. It puts them in proximity to authority and
teaches them how and when to subordinate themselves. It
rewards pragmatic, goal-directed habits of mind. It teaches
people to be aware of subtle status cues and social hierarchies.
More than anything else, it creates a miniature social world
that feels separate and distinct from the world outside the
organization. To step into that world is like crossing over into
Narnia through the wardrobe, only instead of talking lions
and white witches there are middle managers, administrative
assistants, and human resources officers.

It is this crossing of an imaginary border, this sense that the
ordinary world has been left behind, that allows employees to
bracket even deeply held moral convictions when they are on
the job. Working in a bureaucratic organization is like becoming naturalized in a new country where everyone subscribes

to a different set of norms and customs. As a former vice president of a large firm told Jackall, "What is right in the corporation is not what is right in a man's home or in his church.
*What's right in the corporation is what the guy above you wants
from you.* That's what morality is in the corporation."[11]

Corporate morality doesn't simply demand loyalty and
obedience, although that is often the end result. According
to Jackall, the bureaucratic order transforms moral concerns
into practical concerns. What looks like a moral question at
home or at church doesn't look like a moral question in the
bureaucracy, where managers must remain vigilant of the
social rules of their corporate world. They must pay close
attention to the status hierarchy, the norms of etiquette, the
needs of their professional network, and the wishes of their
superiors. When whistleblowers emerge in the bureaucratic
order, they don't look like principled moral dissidents. They
look like disruptive loners who won't play by the rules.

Jackall describes the case of a would-be whistleblower
called Brady, an Englishman working in an American firm.
Brady was a "chartered public accountant," a profession with
considerably more prestige than its American counterpart
and one in which Brady took no small measure of pride. In the
course of his duties as a corporate vice president, Brady came
across a series of serious financial crimes that ultimately led
to the very top of the corporation: bribery, graft, a slush fund,
and falsified records. Like Pesando, Brady attempted to deal
with the issue internally. He escalated his concerns. He went
through the prescribed channels. He spoke to trusted allies.
And like Pesando, Brady was eventually fired.

Here is how Brady described his reasons for continuing to
press his concerns, despite all signs that he would fail:

So what I am saying is that at bottom, I was in jeopardy of violating my professional code. And I feel that

you have to stick up for that. If your profession has standing, it has that standing because someone stood up for it. If the SEC had come in and done an analysis and then went into the details of the case and put me up on the stand and asked me—What is your profession? Was this action right or wrong? Why did you do it then? I would really be in trouble . . . with myself most of all. I am frightened of losing respect, my self-respect in particular. And since that was tied with my respect for my profession, the two things were joined together. I had such a fear of losing that because of my high respect for it.[12]

Self-respect, an ethical code, and concern about public exposure: if you were looking for a case study in honor and dissent, you could scarcely do better. Yet the corporate managers to whom Jackall presented this case didn't see Brady's action in this way at all. They saw it as a practical failure, devoid of any ethical content. In their view, Brady violated the fundamental rules of bureaucratic life. Everyone who works in a corporate setting knows that your job is not to insist on reporting something against the wishes of your boss. Nor is financial misconduct serious enough to warrant a fight. Every company engages in financial sleight of hand, they argued; slush funds, bribes, and doctored invoices are just a fact of corporate life. Brady's private moral code was totally irrelevant. In their view, it was disingenuous for him to insist on the dictates of professional ethics. Nobody gets to be a corporate vice president without making a few moral concessions.

More than anything else, Brady's actions disrupted the social world of the corporation. He broke the unwritten rules. "What it comes down to is that his moral code made other people uncomfortable," one executive said. "He threatened their position."[13] To this executive, it was obvious that Brady was destined to lose this battle from the beginning. He was an evangelist, and even if he was right about the financial misconduct, no manager wants to work with an evangelist.

John Pesando is a quiet man, but it is easy to imagine how uncomfortable he made his colleagues at the Hutch. When he objected to Protocol 126, he violated one of the central social rules of bureaucratic organizations. No wonder he found himself frozen out. "Anxiety is endemic to anyone who works in a corporation," one manager told Jackall.[14] The anxiety comes not just from the fear of failure, but the realization that success requires such vigilant self-control. "Team play" means paying careful attention to social cues and masking your own emotion behind an agreeable smile. Group consensus is the key. Team players must align themselves with the dominant ideology of the moment. They must track its changes carefully. They can't be pushy or outspoken. They have to know when to back off. No evangelists, no crusaders, no prima donnas.

No one enjoys thinking of themselves as silent bystanders to profound wrongdoing. But many of us can probably remember a time when someone insisted on taking action about an issue they found morally outrageous but which failed to move us in the same way. These people usually don't seem heroic. They seem sanctimonious and accusatory. The louder they shout, the more irritating they become. Most annoying of all is their expectation that we will join their moral crusade. It is like listening to the worst kind of sermon, delivered in person by an indignant fundamentalist. These people make us uncomfortable. They make us angry. And they make us even more uncomfortable and angry when they're right.

In Jackall's view, most managers eventually confront a version of the dilemma Brady faced: a clash between the aspects of their self-image that they value and the demands of the social world in which they work. A manager who strongly identifies with the values of honesty and friendship in the outside world will be challenged by a bureaucratic order that consists of ongoing struggles for power and status. A manager who believes in an ethos of egalitarianism will struggle with a corporate culture in which superiors routinely take credit for the work of their subordinates. Unlike Brady, however, most of these managers find some kind of accommodation.

Familiar to most whistleblowers, perhaps especially Pesando, is the way managers deal with the colleague who has failed. That person is isolated and quarantined. The cause of failure doesn't have to be whistleblowing. It doesn't even need to be a moral dispute. It might be a change of upper management or simply bad luck. Whatever the reason, the bureaucratic order has no place for mercy. No one wants to be held responsible for failure, and no one wants to be associated with a person who has failed. As one manager put it, "What we do essentially when someone fails is to put him in a little boat, tow it out to sea, and cut the rope. And we never think about him again."[15]

• • •

Pesando admits he was angry when he was fired. "I had been very badly treated," he says. "When I left the Hutch, I thought I had been disgustingly treated." Yet Protocol 126 was still a mystery to him. Pesando says he just couldn't understand why researchers with such sterling academic credentials would insist on pushing forward with this lethal study. One day in 1991, at the downtown public library in Seattle, Pesando pulled down from the shelf a book by Grant Fjermedal called *Magic Bullets*.[16] And when he read it, the scales fell from his eyes.

Magic Bullets was not supposed to be a work of investigative journalism. It was marketed as a gripping tour of swashbuckling scientific heroism. The cover promises an introduction to "the most exciting adventure in the annals of modern medicine: the coming revolution in cancer therapy." The "magic bullets" of the title are monoclonal antibodies. Fjermedal, a Seattle-based science writer, traveled to cancer centers at Johns Hopkins, Stanford, Harvard, and other universities where he interviewed leading antibody researchers. For the first three quarters of the book, his tone is admiring, even celebratory. Then he made an unsettling visit to the Hutch.

What led Fjermedal to the Hutch was the prospectus for a biotechnology company called Genetic Systems. There he saw that Robert Nowinski, one of the leaders of Genetic Systems, was a former faculty member at the Hutch. The prospectus also listed John Hansen as a principal shareholder with 215,000 shares of stock valued at $1,750,000. Don Thomas, listed as a member of the Genetic Systems scientific advisory board, owned 100,000 shares. Fjermedal was stunned by these arrangements. They looked like egregious conflicts of interest. Fjermedal made an appointment with Bob Day, the director of the Hutch, to ask for an explanation.

Day was evasive. He claimed not to know financial details. He bobbed and weaved, dodging one question after another. The longer Day avoided his questions, the more frustrated Fjermedal became. "This does not sound very diplomatic," Fjermedal told Day, "but I think it appears kind of cheap and sleazy for scientists to be supported by taxpayers at an institution like this, and then to be a millionaire across town at a private company."[17] He compared the situation to journalism. "In the writing of this book, people have asked me, 'Have you bought any stock in these high-tech companies?' The last thing on my mind would be to buy stock in a company I was writing about, because I would see that as a conflict of interest. And now I am finding these researchers who have enormous holdings, and I just think that it isn't correct."[18]

When Fjermedal published *Magic Bullets* in 1984, the structure of American biomedical research was undergoing a major financial shift. The late 1970s and early 1980s had seen the convergence of biotechnology and venture capital with start-ups such as Genentech, Amgen, and Genzyme. A 1980 US Supreme Court decision, *Diamond v. Chakrabarty*, permitted scientists to patent new life-forms. That same year, the US Congress passed the Bayh–Dole Act, which encouraged universities to profit from the results of federally funded research conducted by their faculty members. Soon pharmaceutical and biotechnology companies would begin outsourcing their clinical trials to for-profit contract research organizations (CROs). Biomedical research was transforming itself from an academic enterprise into a profit-driven, multinational business.

With these changes had come alarming new threats to the rights and welfare of research subjects. It had always been assumed that the main threat to subjects came from scientific ambition. Critics worried that researchers might be tempted to take ethical shortcuts in pursuit of promotion, tenure, and academic fame. Yet once it became possible for researchers to reap enormous financial profits from a successful research study, another temptation was added to the mix. Successful researchers could become rich.

John Pesando discovered *Magic Bullets* four years after he lost his job. When he reached the chapter about the Hutch, he was floored. "My eyes just popped out of my head when I was reading this," he says. The money that Genetic Systems was making from monoclonal antibodies was shared not just with the Hutch but with its researchers. This meant that the Hutch and its researchers had a financial stake in the success of Protocol 126. To Pesando, this could explain why the study continued so long despite so many deaths. Pesando thought, "My God, I'd never put the money together as being any significant part of all this." He resolved to tell others what he knew.

Pesando started by writing letters. At first he wrote anonymously, worried that word might get back to his new employer. But his anonymous letters got no response. So Pesando started signing his name to the letters, along with his credentials. That didn't work either. "I wrote to Congress, reporters, everyone else—again, complete lack of interest," he says. "I used to send documents. A good chunk of the evidence I had was the really incriminating stuff." Pesando estimates he sent off at least seventy letters. Only rarely did he even get an acknowledgment. "I wasted a lot of postage," he says.

One agency that eventually agreed to meet with Pesando was the state's medical licensing board. Licensing boards handle disciplinary complaints, usually about substance abuse problems or physicians who are having sex with their patients. "I met with two guys—a physician's assistant and a retired or semiretired physician," Pesando says. "And they listened. 'Politely' is probably the best way to describe it." Pesando says neither of them shared his moral outrage. "When the meeting was over, the assistant—who was clearly the 'worker bee,' so to speak—said to me, 'You should get a life.'"

In May 1993, two years after Pesando began his letter-writing campaign, he finally got the attention of an agency with the authority to act. The federal Office for the Protection from Research Risks (OPRR) started an investigation of the Hutch. Created in 1972 and housed in the National Institutes of Health, OPRR was the primary agency in charge of policing abuses of human research subjects. (In 2000, OPRR was moved from the NIH to the Department of Health and Human Services and renamed the Office for Human Research Protection.) If an IRB was failing to do its job, it was the responsibility of OPRR to investigate.

The OPRR investigation should have marked the point at which the walls of Jericho started to crumble. The agency investigated Protocol 126 for nearly two and a half years. It was given access to much of the written evidence that the *Seattle Times* used to build its damning case against the Hutch six years later. Yet when the agency finally issued a letter in the autumn of 1995, it gave the Hutch a near-total exoneration. It called Pesando's allegations "unsubstantiated" and declared that the agency would not second-guess the IRB.[19] Pesando was devastated. He calls the investigation a farce. "Their job is not to protect patients," he says. "It's to protect the institution."

Yet Pesando did not give up. He kept writing letters, one of which eventually got the attention of reporters at the *Seattle Times*. The *Seattle Times* reporters launched an investigation in which they conducted over one hundred interviews and reviewed approximately ten thousand pages of documents.[20] Among their targets were the financial arrangements between the Hutch and Genetic Systems. According to the *Seattle Times*, a licensing deal for monoclonal antibodies produced at the Hutch had made rich men of Don Thomas and John Hansen when Genetic Systems was bought by Bristol Myers Squibb. Those arrangements had begun to look even more tawdry in 1999, when David Blech, the venture capitalist who founded Genetic Systems at the age of twenty-four, was convicted of securities fraud.[21]

The *Seattle Times* series was published in March 2001, fourteen years after Pesando had lost his job and a decade after he started writing letters. The title of the series was "Uninformed Consent." For a time, it looked as if the series might have an impact. It was short-listed for a Pulitzer Prize and won quite a few awards for journalistic excellence, including the George Polk Award for Medical Reporting, a Goldsmith Prize for Investigative Reporting, the Newspaper Guild's Heywood Broun Award, and the Associated Press Managing Editors Public Service Award. The series also prompted a number of families who had lost loved ones in Protocol 126 to file lawsuits against the Hutch. The jury trial began in February of 2004.

Once again, however, the walls of Jericho held firm. From the very beginning, the families faced long odds, simply because lawsuits about research studies are notoriously difficult to win. Their case was hobbled even further when, midway through the trial, the judge excluded financial conflicts of interests from consideration. In the end, the case turned on the question of informed consent. And despite the testimony of the families, the jury concluded that the subjects had been properly informed. Tom Dreiling, an attorney for the families, said he was shocked by the verdict. "I can't quite believe that 12 reasonable people would reach this conclusion."[22]

In its coverage of the trial, the *Seattle Times* devoted a brief article to Pesando's testimony. "After two days of stoic and at times technical testimony, Dr. John Pesando started to cry," the article began.[23] What brought Pesando to tears was the memory of trying in vain to convince Bob Day to suspend Protocol 126. Day had refused to stop the study, but as a compromise, he had promised that the researchers would no longer enroll patients likely to survive with conventional treatment. That was a promise that Day failed to keep, and patients had died as a result. "These were ethical men. We trusted them," Pesando testified. "When they told us they were going to do something, we assumed that they had done it."[24]

According to Jim Pesando, John's younger brother, no one in the family knew about John's struggle until the *Seattle Times* published its report. That John had kept the conflict to himself was not unusual. "John plays his cards close to the vest," Jim says. But he was not surprised to see John taking up the cause of the victims. That action was totally consistent with the person he had known all his life. "Our family was proud of what he did," Jim says. What Jim remembers even more vividly is the phone call he got from John several years later, informing him that the lawsuit filed against the Hutch had failed. The anguish in John's voice was heartbreaking.

. . .

Defeated whistleblowers need a story that explains their failure without damaging their moral integrity. The story Pesando tells is one about the power that social institutions exert on the public mind. He believes that whistleblowers fail because most people have a deep need to trust in authority. Anyone who tells them that their leaders can't be believed will get a rude welcome. "Society is afraid of anything that challenges their faith in the system and their need for faith in the system," he says. Just as people need to trust government officials, air traffic controllers, and civil engineers, they need to trust doctors, nurses, and researchers. "Our whole society is built on trust. And when the whistleblower comes along and says some of this trust is misplaced, we don't want to believe it. We don't want to hear it. Because most of us couldn't do anything about it anyhow," he says. "Anyone who complains about anything must by definition be wrong, because we live in a perfect society. So, they must be the imperfection, not society."

Although I listen politely, my initial reaction is skepticism. I came of political age during the Watergate scandal. I can't remember a time when most people I knew trusted the government. Over the course of my adult life, I have seen public trust in virtually every American institution crumble away: the justice system, the church, the press, universities, the police. If anything, it feels as if trust has disappeared completely. As we speak, the entire country is awash in paranoid conspiracy theories and political propaganda. Listening to Pesando explain his theory of naive American complacency feels like listening to a crackly radio broadcast from the Eisenhower administration.

As our conversation progresses, however, I gradually come to hear Pesando's message differently. It sounds less like a diagnosis of American society than a conversation with himself as a younger man. "Growing up in a small town, I grew up very trusting of other people and of authority," Pesando says. He was raised in Brampton, Ontario, the oldest of four children. His father was an engineer who worked on military planes. His grandparents, who were both born in Italy, lived in another small town with a large Italian community, most of whom came from the same part of Italy. "We had picnics every Sunday, thirty or forty people," he says. Pesando describes the community of his childhood as nurturing and supportive. "People were good until proven otherwise," he says. "One reason it took so long for me to understand what was going on at the Hutch was I just couldn't believe people would behave this way."

When the company where Pesando's father worked was shut down in 1959, the family moved to Lexington, Massachusetts, where his father had found a new position working on the Saturn rocket program. Pesando was fourteen years old, and the transition from small-town Ontario was rocky. He succeeded academically, however, and was eventually accepted to Harvard University. Although Pesando was gifted at science, he was also drawn to the humanitarian ethos of medicine. "I went into medicine to make it a better place," he says. "I would have gone into the Peace Corps. That's just my value system from my formative years." Pesando's brother, Jim, told me much the same. "John was always a do-gooder," he says.

The political scientist Fred Alford describes the prototypical whistleblower as an idealist who comes late to the cynicism that most of us learn very early on. Unlike most people, who are used to the darker side of human behavior, whistleblowers are genuinely shocked when they discover dishonesty, greed, or corruption. They naively assume that if they blow the whistle, others will be just as outraged as they are. They might even imagine they'll be thanked. And when they lose their jobs and find themselves abandoned by their colleagues, it comes as an existential blow even more staggering than the wrongdoing itself. Alford writes, "The greatest shock is what the whistleblower learns about the world—that nothing he or she believed was true."[25]

Yet if becoming a whistleblower requires a certain naivete, then surviving the experience demands a hard shell of cynicism. Pesando admits that his experience at the Hutch has left some calluses. "I've certainly become a lot more cynical. My wife would be the first one to say that," he says. "I look at the world with a different perspective. I was quite frankly naive and trusting, as I suppose most of us are when we're young. You believe in your government, your institutions. You believe in your leaders, professionally and otherwise. And you need grounds to believe that you shouldn't."

If Pesando once had any idealism about academic medicine, little trace of it remains now. He sees very little in academic medicine to admire. "I think academics brings out some of the worst in terms of behavior, because the behavior required to survive in academic medicine is predatory," he says. "You can't reform it; you can just escape it." And academic medicine tends to attract those for whom a knife in the back is second nature, he tells me. "There are so many back rooms in academics—promotions, space allotments, students, access, grants. You can get stabbed in the back indirectly by a friend of a friend who reviews your grant or sits on the committee and says, you know, this doesn't quite make the pay line. So I think people are excessively fearful. Perhaps they're aware they are vulnerable. Or maybe they're a little paranoid. But as the chairman of Intel said, 'Only the paranoid survive.'"

Pesando was unprepared for the level of savagery he found in the field of oncology. "You sort of figure if you're going into cancer medicine, we are all united here—fighting the Germans on the front lines, so to speak. And in fact, you know, taking care of your own interests was the first priority. For most of

the colleagues that I met—not all, there were some naive ide-
alists like myself—but by and large, treating cancer and saving
patients was a secondary purpose," he says. The first priority
was career success. "People perceive the world as being filled
with finite resources, and if you get something, I don't. That
seems to be the rules of the game. And I cannot say everybody
in medicine feels that way, but those who stay in academic
medicine have to prepare to play by those perceived rules," he
says. "So, they are particularly, what's the word that I'm looking for?" Pesando pauses for a second. "Sociopathic?" I say.
"Yes, sociopathic," he replies.

I ask Pesando if he feels ashamed of the medical profession.
He hesitates. "This goes beyond medicine. Medicine per se has
no power," he says. "Medicine couldn't put a stop to what was
going on at the Fred Hutch, for example." This remark puzzles
me. Don Thomas was a physician. So was Bob Day, the director, as well as Paul Martin and John Hansen, the investigators
on Protocol 126. Surely, they could have stopped the study. I
point out to Pesando that the medical profession is supposed
to be self-policing. "The honor system," he says, laughing.
"Well, when there is no honor." He pauses. "I've never been a
believer in an honor system."

It's tough to get a handle on what Pesando does believe in.
He doesn't speak of shame, guilt, or self-respect. He resists
any talk of honor, and he says he has no heroes. When I ask
whether his experience at the Hutch changed the way he
raised his daughter, he replies, "I don't think so." I ask if he
had a religious upbringing. "Yes and no. My father raised us
as Catholics," he says. "At the age of twelve or thirteen, I basically said, 'This is horseshit.'" At every turn he resists my
efforts to dig deeper into his moral sensibility. I ask about the
values he inherited from his parents growing up. "Virtually no
feedback," he replies. When I ask if he feels proud of the moral
stand he took at the Hutch, he responds with an emphatic no.

Nor does he feel ashamed. "I did what I had to do," he says. "That's all. It comes with the territory."

Yet Pesando is steadfast in his moral convictions. For him, the matter was simple. He knew that patients were dying. "And I felt a moral obligation to do whatever I could to prevent it," he says. At the Hutch, he felt complicit in the harm. "To sit and watch somebody getting hurt, it's equivalent to hurting them if I don't do something about it. Or try to do something about it. That's the best I can do to explain it," he says. "I'd like to think I've never hurt another person in this life, at least not deliberately, and that's just who I am."

The phrase "that's just who I am" is revealing. It suggests principled action set into motion almost without conscious decision. It is a phrase many whistleblowers settle on as a final explanation for their actions. *I did what I did because I am the kind of person who could not do otherwise.* What makes Pesando different is the way he judges that person. Pesando speaks of his younger self less as a moral exemplar than as a dupe, the unwitting mark in a big con. People who remain silent in the face of wrongdoing are not cowards; they just have enough brains to avoid being suckered. "I say that with great pain, because obviously I was not so bright," Pesando says. He doesn't seem bitter or angry anymore. He just sounds defeated.

Defeat means sacrificing a career for nothing. Pesando spent the first half of adult life training to be a cancer researcher and the second half reviewing disability claims. Merely seeing the wrongdoing at the Hutch exposed gives Pesando no satisfaction. "I mean, if something had been accomplished, if the rules had been changed, if the government regulations had reflected—filling in those gaps in the regulations that people routinely ignore to my knowledge to this day—then I would have a sense of accomplishment," he says. "As it is, I can point to nothing specifically that has changed since I was there." As for whether he would do the same thing again, Pesando can't say. "If you thought you would do some good—even if you thought you'd take a personal hit—maybe you would. But in the case of the Hutch, I'm not sure we did anything good of long-lasting value."

Pesando and I are sitting outside on a bench again, this one outside a building that used to house the Hutch. I talked him into meeting me here in the hope that it might jog some memories. "My office was in the old nursing building," he says, pointing across the way. "That's gone." Pesando swings around on the bench and pulls up his legs, crossing them like a Boy Scout. For a man in his mid-seventies, he is surprisingly fit. Two decades ago, the Hutch moved across town to an upscale waterfront campus that Pesando has never visited. When I went to see the new campus, I texted Pesando a photo. Perched on a pedestal was a bust of Bob Day, the former president of the Hutch. "Who says crime doesn't pay?" Pesando responded.

Pesando is a private person by nature. He doesn't share a lot about his personal life. But waging a private moral battle against a powerful institution can be very lonely even in the best of circumstances. Not many people are psychologically equipped to survive such a solitary fight. Pesando says he always felt like an outsider at the Hutch, with no real friends or close colleagues. Even the colleagues who seemed to agree that Protocol 126 was an unethical study were unwilling to take any significant action to stop it. Until the *Seattle Times* series came out, Pesando didn't even discuss the issue with his friends or family members. He admits this was hard. "You've got nobody to bounce things off of," he says. "What should I do? Is this really worth pursuing? Am I missing something?" I tell Pesando that a battle so solitary seems almost unendurable. "Well, it became increasingly stressful," he says. "As you might imagine. It became very clear within six months that this was not conducive to my career."

Pesando does not embrace the term "whistleblower." "When I hear 'whistleblower,' I hear 'snitch,'" he says. "People look at you differently. It's like, 'None of us is perfect. And if you're famous for blowing the whistle, maybe you'll blow some whistle in my direction.' You're damaged goods." Pesando says he didn't want to be named in the *Seattle Times* series. He relented only because he was told that going on the record publicly was necessary to give the story credibility. "I did not want it," he says. "No way. Fame? This is not fame."

Pesando doesn't seem prickly or defensive, yet his self-assessment is so relentlessly critical that I find myself arguing with him, trying to make the case that he should feel proud of following his conscience. "Is there no nobility in trying to do the right thing?" I ask. To which Pesando replies, "In our society, are you kidding?" To me it seems that Pesando has set an impossibly high standard for moral decency. Sometimes you try to do the right thing but fail, I tell him. Not everything is within our control. Flailing around for an example of a noble failure, I come up with Claus von Stauffenberg, the German army officer who tried unsuccessfully to assassinate Hitler. Pesando concedes, "I would make an exception for that." But he sees his own failure as different.

"Maybe if society thought I did the right thing—if others, other than myself, thought that it was a worthwhile activity," Pesando says. "Most people don't. They don't know why you failed to accomplish anything." According to Pesando, most people in Seattle are totally unaware of what happened at the Hutch. "They don't know that I was the whistleblower. They don't know that there was a newspaper series or a trial or even any facts. They have absolutely no clue, including my neighbors," he says. I ask if there is no consolation in knowing in his heart that he did the right thing. "There's some solace, but not a lot," Pesando says. "Do I get up in the morning and say, 'You did the right thing, by God?' No, I don't."

• • •

Our trip home from Seattle is much easier than our journey west. Rain has brought the wildfires under control. We decide to stop for a night in Idaho at the Lower Stanley Country Store and Motel, deep in the Sawtooth Mountains. In the afternoon we hike the Redfish Lake Trail. Along the trail are thousands of downed trees, gray and brittle, as if a giant box of wooden matches has been emptied in the forest. The wildlife is almost tame, deer staring at us not 20 feet away, chipmunks daring us to do something. Yellow aspens shimmer in the late afternoon sun. Their leaves look like the golden chocolate coins we used to put in the children's stockings at Christmas.

When we get back to the motel, Ina fries some potatoes and onions in the kitchenette. I open a beer, sit back on the bed, and think about John Pesando. His long struggle against the Hutch seems so lonely. If only he had been joined in his struggle by one true friend. If only he had been vindicated by just one oversight body or court. I wonder if anyone else has ever tried to convince Pesando that he had acted honorably. Dr. King may have thought that the moral arc of the universe bends toward justice, but King never had to argue with John Pesando. I can imagine Pesando responding modestly with a nihilistic joke, his eyes cast downward. I wish I could convince him that his struggle had made a difference.

As I look back over the *Seattle Times* series, I see that Pesando was not the only physician at the Hutch who was skeptical of Protocol 126. Another critic was Rainer Storb, one of the founders of the Hutch and an expert on graft-versus-host disease. Storb said he could see all along that Protocol 126 was failing. "It was becoming evident on the wards that, you know, something's really fishy here," Storb said. "You have to have a very keen eye and bring the whole thing to a screeching halt if something goes wrong."[26] Storb told the *Seattle Times* that he stated his opposition to Protocol 126 repeatedly at staff meetings. I decide to call Storb when I get back to Minnesota.

At the age of eighty-five, Storb is still the head of the Transplantation Biology Program at the Hutch and holds the Milton B. Rubin Family Endowed Chair. When I reach him by phone, I find him friendly, open, and disarmingly blunt in his assessment of Protocol 126. "I thought it was outright stupid, really, to T-deplete," Storb says. His own research on GVHD at the time suggested that T cell depletion would fail. Storb also felt it was a mistake for the Protocol 126 researchers to move so quickly from animals to human trials. "That stuff that was done in humans, I would have done in experimental animals," Storb says. "That was my approach, always. I never introduced anything in the clinic until I had years and years of animal experimentation done and was really absolutely sure that things worked like this and could be safely transferred to humans. But that was not done in this case."

Beginning in the mid-1970s, Storb says, he established a Wednesday morning meeting to discuss GVHD. He describes the meetings as "free-for-alls" in which weighty scientific issues could be freely debated. Don Thomas was a regular attendee. Storb remembers leveling harsh criticism at Protocol 126 at those meetings. "I said things very clearly," he says. "I think something like, 'It seems we have killed enough patients by now. We should really move on.'" At one point Storb suggested abandoning Protocol 126 in favor of another GVHD study that looked exciting but did not involve monoclonal antibodies. But Protocol 126 was continued, Storb says, because Thomas was behind it.

Equally disturbing to Storb were the financial relationships between the researchers and Genetic Systems. Storb says he knew nothing about those entanglements until much later. "I was really disappointed in Don. I mean, I'd never expected that from Don Thomas," Storb says. "I thought he was above that kind of stuff, basically." Storb tells me he has always stayed away from industry relationships. His research funding has come from the federal government.

I am a little surprised by how forthright Storb is. I had expected a little defensiveness or at least an excuse on behalf of the institution. But Storb is relentlessly critical. "If I had run a protocol like that, I would feel terrible," he says. "Just because I'm not only a researcher but also a physician, and the reason for me coming to Seattle was that I wanted to do something that eventually might be able to help patients." He is grateful he was never faced with the decision whether to enroll any of his own patients in Protocol 126. "I would have counseled against it, to be quite honest right now," he says. "I just couldn't in good conscience have put a patient on that protocol." When I ask him if he thinks the families of the research subjects who died in Protocol 126 deserved an apology from the Hutch, Storb says yes.

What I am trying to reconcile is the difference between Rainer Storb and John Pesando. If Storb believed that Protocol 126 was killing patients, why didn't he do more to stop it? "I'm sure I talked about it at meetings, when meeting colleagues from other institutions," Storb says, pointing out that many other institutions were doing research on T cell depletion at the time. I press Storb further by email later, asking if he had ever considered taking his concerns to an oversight body such as OPRR or the FDA. He says no. "The thought of going, say, to the FDA did not occur to me," Storb says. "I believed that continuously raising my concerns about the trial at the weekly meeting and the review of each new trial version by the IRB were enough. Also, I had two competing trials of my own going at the same time. That fact alone made even my almost weekly questioning of 126 appear biased."

In *Moral Mazes*, Robert Jackall explains that the cardinal virtue for corporate managers is discretion. Only by remaining circumspect and diplomatic can they establish faith with others. "Nobody would ever consciously plan to do something that would endanger people," a manager said. "But when things happen, well, you cover for yourself and your company."[27] Storb reminds me of that manager. Raising his concerns externally would have violated institutional norms of discretion and solidarity. Storb says that faculty members at the Hutch must generate a quarter of their own salaries through grants, most of them collaborations with other faculty members. "It would have been difficult to violate the spirit of collaboration by going outside of the Hutch to complain about a colleague's trial," Storb says. He is right, of course. It would have been very difficult. Yet that is what the honor code requires.

When litigation was brought by the families of subjects against the Hutch in 2004, Storb was placed in the uncomfortable position of being called to give testimony. According to the *Seattle Times*, Storb testified that he had serious doubts about Protocol 126. But he also cautioned that such reservations are commonplace in the scientific community. "Unfortunately, in science, many of the hypotheses that one forms later turn out to be wrong," Storb said. "We all had doubts about each others' approaches. You're sort of pushing the envelope, and you don't know where you're going to be in the end."[28] Storb told the court he would have been willing to enroll patients in Protocol 126, despite his reservations.

In the end, what set Pesando apart from Storb and everyone else at the Hutch was his willingness to go to authorities outside the institution rather than simply expressing his opposition internally. I ask Storb what he thinks of Pesando's decision. "I think John was crushed by not being promoted," Storb says. "So, he may just be still hurt and he still may be driven by this combination of personal failure and of not being promoted and seeing the Hutch as a kind of enemy figure. I really think it's a deep-seated psychological issue with him," he says. "John is a bit of a tragic figure."

I ask Storb if he thinks Pesando might have acted for conscientious reasons. Is it not possible that Pesando was genuinely troubled by the fact that subjects were dying unnecessarily? "I don't know," Storb says, struggling as he considers the question. "I don't know," he says again. "He was a strange character. He was always so secretive." It sounds as if Storb has never even considered the possibility that Pesando had acted honorably. "I don't know if I really can say whether he was, because of ethics, upset about it," Storb finally says. "Could be. I can't really say."

• • •

On the top floor of my house, in the room known as the Institute for Nixon Studies, there is a framed jigsaw puzzle of a postage stamp bearing the likeness of Richard Nixon. The stamp was issued in 1995, one year after Nixon's death and twenty-one years after he resigned in disgrace. It is an American tradition to honor presidents in this way after they die, no matter how shameful or politically disastrous their record in office. Somehow this honor seems fitting for Nixon, a man who kept clawing his way back to power in a cut-throat arena that rewards treachery and duplicity. On the stamp there is just a hint of a smile on Nixon's face.

Don Thomas was never featured on a postage stamp, but he did win a Nobel Prize. The Nobel Assembly at the Karolinska Institute honored Thomas in 1990, citing his achievements in bone marrow transplantation. Protocol 126 had been long forgotten by the time Thomas died in 2012. His obituaries did not mention the controversy, though they noted his determination in the face of failure. The *New York Times* said that many physicians in the 1950s had abandoned the idea of bone marrow transplantation for fear that it would never be safe enough to be practical. "Dr. Thomas persevered, despite numerous failures and the criticism that he was exposing his patients to undue risks."[29]

It can't be easy to take on a Nobel laureate, much less do battle with him in the public arena. As I think about Pesando's long struggle, one detail keeps nagging at me. I simply can't understand how the Office for Protection from Research Risks exonerated the Hutch. The name on the OPRR letter, Tom Puglisi, is familiar to me. Puglisi was compliance director at a time when the agency built a well-earned reputation for vigilance on behalf of research subjects. In the late 1990s, OPRR shut down federally funded research at eight major medical research institutions for failure to properly oversee their research programs. Puglisi was one of three OPRR officials whose photograph had appeared in a 1999 *US News and World Report* article: fierce looks on their faces, their arms folded like bouncers.[30] Even his name sounds aggressive. Did Puglisi really believe the Hutch was blameless? I decide to track him down.

"I'm not proud of having signed this letter. I'll be totally honest with you," Puglisi tells me when I reach him by phone. Although Puglisi did not recall the Hutch case when I first contacted him, his memory came back when I sent him the *Seattle Times* series and the documents from the OPRR office. His self-assessment is disarmingly honest. OPRR got the decision wrong. "So, what did you say, that we blew it? I think you're right," he says.

Puglisi agrees with Pesando that the subjects in Protocol 126 were misled. The researchers did not properly inform the subjects about the risks of the study or that a second transplant almost always failed. "That's totally, totally egregious. And why we didn't pursue the issue of truly informed consent mystifies me," he says. Nor can Puglisi understand how the agency glossed over the failure of the research team to inform

the IRB when subjects died. "To me that is the most concerning thing about what we did, or didn't do, that we didn't
push hard about. I don't know where it was in the letter, but
I remember when I read it the other day thinking, "God, how
mealy-mouthed can you get?"

While Puglisi makes no excuses for the OPRR decision, he
does offer some explanations. One was how short-staffed the
agency was at the time. "I wish we could have conducted more
site visits, but we didn't have the staff power and there was no
way we were going to get the staff power," Puglisi says. Another
problem was a matter of jurisdiction. "The biggest stumbling
block, I think, was the fact that we really didn't have oversight
authority over conflict of interest," Puglisi says. "The conflict-
of-interest guidelines at that point were very, very vague. I
don't know if I have the timeline exactly right, but I think the
policy then was you had to have a policy. That's about it."

Puglisi seems embarrassed by the OPRR decision. He says
that someone else in his office wrote the determination letter
exonerating the Hutch. "I mean, I signed it, and I take responsibility for it, but I clearly didn't write it because it's not my
writing style," Puglisi says. "But nevertheless, I should have
pushed much harder in that case. I absolutely would go on
record—would not mind being quoted—saying that I should
have pushed harder in that case. Because I think there is a
'there' there that we just maybe didn't want to see."

After Puglisi and I hang up, I call Pesando. It is Canadian
Thanksgiving and Pesando greets me cheerfully. He seems
very happy to hear about Puglisi's reversal. While his cynicism
is undiminished, there is a lightness in his voice that I hadn't
heard before. His laugh is louder, and it comes more often.
He thanks me for calling Puglisi. "Even though nothing good
came out of it, it's at least good to know that people are aware
that things weren't quite what they should be," he says.

I don't know if Puglisi's opinion will change the story

Pesando tells himself. The walls of Jericho never fell; the Hutch is still thriving. But at least it provides some external affirmation that Pesando was right. Back in Seattle, Pesando and I talked about how hard it is to wage a solitary battle that nobody else thinks worth fighting. "What kind of preparation can there be in life for this kind of traumatic event? It's almost like serving in the military in the front lines," he said. "Honestly, it just wears you down." It's not just that you need help or support. It is also a matter of confidence in your own moral judgment. It takes strength to hold fast to your principles when you are completely alone. Pesando said, "At some point you have to question your values and say, 'Why am I the only person in the room who thinks this way?'"

CHAPTER 5

Cincinnati

As a rule, I'm reluctant to ask for directions until absolutely necessary. But after twenty minutes in the University of Cincinnati Medical Center, it's clear that without help, I'll never find what I'm looking for. Somewhere on the grounds of this hospital is a memorial. I don't know what it looks like or where exactly it is located, but it is dedicated to the victims of a deadly series of total body irradiation experiments conducted here in the 1960s. In June 2017, however, it appears that nobody at the hospital has ever heard of it. One clerk tries to direct me to the Department of Radiology. Others just shake their heads and look blank. Eventually, the word "radiation" unlodges an idea. A clerk makes a phone call to Nuclear Medicine, where she finally finds success. A young woman there knows exactly the memorial I am looking for and would be happy to take me to it. She works at the Eugene Saenger Radioisotope Laboratory.

The Eugene Saenger Radioisotope Laboratory is the very clinic where the radiation experiments were planned and executed. Saenger was a renowned radiologist and specialist in nuclear medicine. From 1960 until 1972, he was funded by the Pentagon to expose nearly ninety vulnerable cancer patients to potentially lethal total body irradiation. The majority of his subjects were poor and Black, and many died soon after they were exposed. The purpose of the experiments was not to cure their cancer. The purpose was to help the Pentagon determine how much radiation American soldiers could withstand in a nuclear attack.[1]

The young woman from the Saenger Laboratory leads me down a series of poorly lit underground corridors. Eventually, we come to a stairwell, and I am led out to an empty courtyard. I look around. All I see is the back wall of a parking garage and some machinery. The courtyard looks like a place where hospital employees might go to sneak a cigarette. "Over here," my friendly guide tells me, pointing to some overgrown shrubbery near the wall of the hospital. "Look in the bushes." Behind the shrubbery I finally see the "memorial." It is a brown metal plaque about 2 feet tall. At the top it says, "In Memoriam Cancer Patients, Radiation Effects Study, 1960–72." Below is a roll call of patient names. At the bottom it reads, "Presented by their families." The "memorial" includes no apology, no expression of gratitude, and no mention of Eugene Saenger. Even if the plaque were not completely obscured by shrubbery, it would have been easy to overlook. The plaque faces the wall of the hospital.

I'm still shaking my head when my guide offers to show me the Saenger Laboratory. Saenger practiced medicine at the University of Cincinnati for over thirty years. When he retired, the College of Medicine awarded him the Daniel Drake Medal, its highest honor, and established an endowment fund in his name.[2] A glass cabinet in the laboratory houses a tribute to him. Some of Saenger's awards are displayed in the cabinet, along with vintage medical instruments, radiology manuals, and a group photo of smiling doctors wearing plaid pants. As I look at the cabinet, I remember that the theologian Stanley Hauerwas once claimed that the modern medical center represents our culture's equivalent of a Gothic cathedral. If Hauerwas is right, then this cabinet is a shrine to a local saint.

For the experimenter, a shrine; for his subjects, a plaque hidden in the shrubbery. Somehow this seems fitting. The public learned of Saenger's radiation experiments in the fall of 1971, roughly the same period as the so-called holy trinity of American research scandals: the Tuskegee syphilis experiment, the Willowbrook hepatitis experiment, and the Jewish Chronic Disease Hospital cancer experiment.[3] Each of those scandals is memorialized in bioethics textbooks and routinely taught to medical students. Yet the Cincinnati radiation experiments are not remembered even in the very hospital where they were carried out.

For nearly fifty years, nobody has worked harder than Martha Stephens to ensure that this would not happen. Stephens is a rare bird: a whistleblower who blew twice. In 1972, when she was a young assistant professor in the University of Cincinnati's English department, Stephens helped expose Saenger's experiments and led the effort to shut them down. Twenty-one years later, after Eileen Welsome, of the *Albuquerque Tribune*, began to unravel the vast scope of secret Cold War radiation experimentation, Stephens stepped forward again. She tracked down the families of the Cincinnati victims and helped them launch a lawsuit. A decade later she published a book about the experiments called *The Treatment: The Story of Those Who Died in the Cincinnati Radiation Tests*. It was in her book that I learned about the memorial, which the hospital erected in the late 1990s to help settle a lawsuit by the victims. Stephens had recommended that the plaque be inscribed with a phrase taken from Shelley's sonnet *Ozymandias*: "Look on my works, ye mighty, and despair."[4]

Unlike many whistleblowers, Stephens didn't simply find herself with inside information about wrongdoing. She knew nothing about the radiation research at her university until she read about it in a newspaper article. But once Stephens learned about the research, she couldn't let it drop. So, she started digging, and then she dug some more, and over time, she had dug so deeply into the walls of secrecy surrounding the experiments that the entire structure collapsed. That's why I've come to Cincinnati to meet her. As I stand in the shrubbery to snap a photo of the plaque, I wonder what Stephens will make of it.

· · ·

To hear Eugene Saenger tell it, the controversy over his work was a hit job by left-wing political crusaders. "The attack came really from people who were unilateral disarmament people," he says. I am watching a videotaped interview produced by the university in 1984.[5] Saenger says that the attacks intensified until they were picked up by Senator Edward Kennedy, a wily Democratic politician with opportunistic motives. "He felt he needed some ammunition to attract the public to see that he was a defender of the poor, the weak and the downtrodden," Saenger explains. Dr. Charles Barrett, one of the interviewers, turns to the camera and says how much he admired the way Saenger responded. "I gained even greater respect for Eugene's character and perseverance in this, because this was like landing a haymaker on somebody who's coming out of a shower," Barrett says, shaking his head. "I mean, it just hit."

Saenger was a true son of Cincinnati. Except for four years as an undergraduate at Harvard and two years in the military, Saenger spent his entire life in the city. He grew up in Cincinnati, went to medical school there, and did his residency training there. His uncle was the first chair of the University of Cincinnati's Department of Radiology. His interest in radiation went back to his time in the Army Medical Corps, where, by his own account, Saenger got an introduction to "bombol-ogy." He was discharged from military service in 1955, but he kept up his military connections for the rest of his career.[6]

As soon as Saenger was discharged, he started working on a research proposal for total-body irradiation. The impe-tus came partly from a colleague in pediatrics who claimed that no radiologist had ever done good research. "That really upset me. That really annoyed me," Saenger said later. "I have never forgotten that. I sort of thought, dammit, I'm going to show people I know how to do something."[7] In 1958, Saenger applied to the Army Surgeon General's office for funding for a study titled "Metabolic Changes in Humans Following Total Body Irradiation." Saenger would later claim it was an appli-cation to study cancer treatment, but that was not true. Its main purpose was to identify a biological "dosimeter," a test that could measure exposure to radiation. From 1960 to 1971, the military gave Saenger over $670,000 in research funding.[8]

Saenger certainly doesn't look like a guilty man in the video. He looks like a distinguished physician in his later years, peer-ing over half-rim glasses, his head slightly cocked, his manner gentle and confident. Saenger makes self-deprecating jokes. When he is complimented, he responds with a rueful smile, glancing modestly at the floor. His explanation of the radia-tion experiments is very convincing. Saenger says he was sim-ply trying to compare the effects of total body irradiation with the effects of chemotherapy in patients with disseminated cancers. The proper authorities had approved all his research when leftist critics falsely accused him of mismanaging Pen-tagon funds. The accusation was investigated by the Govern-ment Accountability Office, which found that not a nickel of Pentagon money was misspent. With that, Senator Kennedy was forced to back off.

Like the best falsehoods, Saenger's account is presented

with such confidence and authority that a casual viewer would have little reason to suspect it was untrue. Saenger's credibility is enhanced by the teasing banter of his two interviewers, both old colleagues from the medical school. In 1984, however, none of the men could know that in ten years Saenger's experiments would be the target of a federal investigation and a lawsuit. As I watch the interview now, with the benefit of hindsight, I'm struck by a comment Saenger makes toward the end, almost as an afterthought. One of the underappreciated keys to his success at the University of Cincinnati, Saenger notes, is that nobody at the medical school ever interfered with his work. He says, "There's an attitude in this medical school that no one is really ever against what you're trying to do."[9]

In the fall of 1971, Martha Stephens was an untenured professor of English at the University of Cincinnati. It was her first academic position after graduate school. Richard Nixon had been in office for nearly two years, and young men were still being drafted to fight in the Vietnam War. Only a year and a half earlier, on the campus of Kent State University, 250 miles north of Cincinnati, the National Guard had opened fire on unarmed protesters, killing four students and injuring another nine. One day in a corridor of McMicken Hall, Stephens was stopped by a colleague in political science who had an article to show her. "We're doing some kind of war research here," he said, handing her a brief article, maybe from the *Village Voice*. The article was about Eugene Saenger and his military radiation experiments. "God, we don't want that on our campus," Stephens said.

It is June 2018, and Stephens and I are sitting together at the dining room table in her house in Paddock Hills, a quiet neighborhood in the northern part of Cincinnati. The room is crowded with books and papers. Stephens is a tiny, slender woman with short gray hair. Like me, she is a Southerner. Stephens grew up in Waycross, Georgia, a little town north of the

Okefenokee Swamp. She has a warm, down-home manner, but she is fierce and outspoken in her political opinions. On the front door of her house is a sign that says, "God is coming and boy, is she pissed." At age eighty-one Stephens has developed a vision problem that requires her to wear large glasses and a visor to shield the light, even indoors. The visors she buys from the Salvation Army and decorates with hand-drawn peace signs and political slogans. When she tells me about her past, she speaks with a lyrical rhythm, repeating phrases like a preacher, her lilt broken up occasionally by hoots of laughter. Her manner and accent sound so much like home that I keep catching myself about to say, "Yes, ma'am."

The story of Saenger's experiments first emerged on October 8, 1971. A front-page headline in the *Washington Post* read, "Pentagon Has Contract to Test Radiation Effect on Humans."[10] According to the *Post*, the purpose of the Cincinnati study was to understand how whole body radiation affected the "combat-readiness" of soldiers on the battlefield. To test the effects of radiation, Saenger recruited patients whose cancer could no longer be helped by surgery. All but three of them were "charity cases," and their average length of schooling was only six years. Saenger did not tell them about the dangerous side effects of total body irradiation. Nor did he mention that the experiments were being conducted for military purposes. Saenger and his junior collaborator, Edward Silberstein, told the *Post* that their aim was to help their patients, but other academic specialists were skeptical. "Nobody to my knowledge is using this (whole body radiation) as a therapeutic measure," a radiologist from Memorial Sloan Kettering Cancer Center said. "It approaches what happens in an atomic accident."

After the *Post* broke the story, the major news outlets jumped into action, as well as international media organizations such as *Stern* and *The Times* of London. A new book by Roger Rapoport, *The Great American Bomb Machine,* out-lined Saenger's work for the Pentagon in even more detail.[11] Scrambling to defend itself, the University of Cincinnati held a press conference. David Logan, a former University of Cincinnati English professor, says the university presented a three-pronged defense: "We didn't do anything wrong; we've never done anything wrong; and we're not going to do it again." Administrators claimed that all Saenger's subjects had been fully informed, that nothing was done in secret, and that the care Saenger gave his subjects far exceeded that of standard practice.

Stephens decided she had to see the radiation study records for herself. One afternoon she drove over to see Dr. Edward Gall, the head of the medical center. Gall turned out to be a shy, pleasant man who politely refused her request to see the records. Stephens, a shy, pleasant woman, politely refused to take no for an answer. "I went back three times," Stephens says, "and the third time, there was a stack of docu-ments on his desk." Gall told her, "Look, I'm going to give you these; I don't think you'll be interested in them. In fact, I'm not sure that anyone who's not in medicine would understand them." Stephens drove back to the English department for a 2 p.m. class and parked. "I pulled those papers out on my lap," she says. "I saw that at the end of each report there were pro-files of the subjects of the research, a page or two for each one. And so, sitting there that day, I saw that some died. They died from what was done to them."

The documents were Saenger's reports to the Department of Defense. "They wanted to find a 'dosimeter,' a dose indi-cator, that could be applied to soldiers in combat to see how much radiation they'd absorbed," Stephens says. "If they've been exposed on the fringes of a bomb, will they get real sick? Will a pilot be able to fly his plane? You wanted to test them right after their exposure. So that's why they irradiated people. They irradiated them, then they tested them. They tested their urine. They tested their blood, their mental condition after irradiation," Stephens says. "They might as well have said, 'We killed this person. Too bad.'"

The symptoms of acute radiation syndrome—nausea, vomiting, fatigue, and weakness—typically begin within hours of radiation exposure. In order to observe these symptoms carefully for his military funders, Saenger had denied most of the patients any medication to relieve their nausea and vomiting for three days.[12] If a patient survived this period, there was usually a latent period of about twenty days, followed by another period of acute illness. This second period was the most dangerous. Patients would often develop fever, abdominal pain, diarrhea, bleeding, and shock. The most serious hazard was infection due to bone marrow suppression, which could easily lead to death.

One of the patients was Katie Dennis, a Black woman in her fifties who had four daughters at home. Dennis was hospitalized for lung cancer when Saenger enrolled her in his experiment. Saenger gave her 250 rads of total body irradiation.[13] "They said that she would moan during the night for medicine," Stephens says. "She would cry out, 'Pain, pain.' Her left leg was hurting so bad. And the nurse would have to say, 'Not time for your medicine yet.' Well, she died seven days after she was irradiated."

Looking back, Stephens identifies that afternoon in her car as the point of no return. If she had simply waited to see how things would play out, she might have forgotten about the experiments. But once she had read the stories of the individual patients, it was impossible to keep quiet. "When I pulled those papers out on my lap, sitting there in my car in front of my hall, as far as I knew, I was probably the only person that had ever read them, other than people in the College of Medicine," Stephens says. "I'll have to tell what I am reading here," she thought. "I can't let this be a secret that only I know."

Stephens was in no position to protest the experiments. She didn't have any background in medicine, much less nuclear medicine or radiology. Nor did she have tenure. Accusing her own university of collaborating with the military to exploit vulnerable cancer patients could ruin her career. What she did have, however, was a small group of like-minded colleagues who opposed the Vietnam War. They called themselves the Junior Faculty Association. The association had been organized in part by Martha's husband, Jerone, a political science professor, to help protect untenured faculty members in their careers—although the word "organized" suggests a degree of order and efficiency that the group never actually had. "I don't remember if you had to join," Martha says. "I don't know that you did. We just called ourselves an association."

In December Stephens wrote a detailed, highly critical report about the experiments based on the documents she had been given. Five or six of her fellow Junior Faculty Association members signed it, and on January 25, 1972, they called a press conference on campus to present the report. Dave Logan read the report out loud. Not many journalists turned up. Most local reporters were off covering a fire at a nursing home. But one reporter in attendance happened to be a stringer for the *Washington Post*. The resulting article, "Faculty Study Hits Whole-Body Radiation Plan," caught the attention of Senator Edward Kennedy, who was preparing hearings on medical experimentation.[14] He submitted both the *Post* article and the JFA report into the Congressional Record.[15]

The report Stephens prepared, "A Report to the Campus Community," is a remarkable document, especially given the period in which it was written. Stephens had no background in medical ethics; in fact, the field was still in its infancy. Yet her report is utterly convincing. She identified three key questions. First, was the study of cancer the main aim of the experiments? Second, what were the risks to the patients? Third, did the patients give their consent to being used as research subjects? Having identified the questions, Stephens carefully dismantled Saenger's justification of the experiments, leaving little doubt that they were morally indefensible.

First, as Stephens pointed out, the written record contained no evidence of any systematic study of cancer. Yet for over a decade Saenger and his team had prepared detailed, painstakingly modified proposals to study the effects of radiation on human physiology. They had published several articles on potential dosimeters and not a single article about the effects of total body irradiation on cancer. Stephens asked, "Is it conceivable that, in an authentic cancer research study, no results would be reported after eleven years and the radiation of 87 patients?"

Second, the risks of the study were terrifying. Nearly a quarter of the subjects died within thirty-eight days of being irradiated. Four died within only ten days. The higher the dose of radiation, the more likely the subjects were to die. These patients were by no means on the verge of death before they were irradiated. Saenger himself described the patients as being in "relatively good health" and said that many were "working daily." As Stephens noted, even if their condition had somehow improved as a result of irradiation, it would have been difficult to tell, because Saenger had failed to use a control group.

Finally, Stephens dispatched with any suggestion that Saenger's subjects had given meaningful informed consent. For the first five years of the study, Saenger used no written consent forms whatsoever. Subjects were simply told (falsely) that the radiation was part of their cancer treatment. In 1965, Saenger began giving patients a short consent form, but it mentioned nothing about the risks of radiation. Five years later, in 1970, a new consent form finally listed the risks of the study, but it identified them as "infection and mild bleeding." Saenger began using a longer form in the spring of 1971, but even at that late date he failed to mention that subjects might die from bone marrow failure.

As impressive as the report was, there was no getting around the fact that it came from a small group of untenured scholars without any medical credentials. Saenger, in contrast, had the backing of the medical establishment and the university. When the American College of Radiology (ACR) appointed an investigative committee led by a friend of Saenger's, the outcome was complete exoneration.[16] The University of Cincinnati launched an internal investigation led by Raymond Suskind, a professor of Environmental Health, that included a member of Saenger's research team as well as four other faculty members who had previously approved the research. Its report was much more critical than that of the ACR, but it concluded that the university should permit Saenger to continue.[17]

In early February 1972, the fate of the radiation experiments was still unclear. Alaska Senator Mike Gravel was asking hard questions, and Senator Edward Kennedy was preparing to hold hearings on medical experimentation. Staff members for Kennedy were pressuring the University of Cincinnati to allow interviews with the subjects or their families, but the university refused, claiming that interviews would violate the patients' privacy. Stephens and her allies still held out hope that Kennedy's Senate hearings would include Saenger's experiments.

Two events brought the controversy to a sputtering end. On February 24, Kennedy and his staff met with university officials and John Gilligan, the Democratic governor of Ohio. Soon after that meeting, Kennedy dropped his efforts to interview patients. When the Senate hearings began, they did not include the Cincinnati experiments. Two months later, as the president of the university, Warren Bennis, was still deciding whether to let the experiments proceed, Saenger signed a new research agreement with the Department of Defense. He had been secretly negotiating the agreement for months. When Bennis learned that Saenger had signed an agreement behind his back, he immediately issued a directive ending all military funding. Saenger tried to get funding from the National Cancer Institute, but in September of 1972, his application was rejected. With that, Saenger's radiation study came to a quiet close.[18]

The absence of a clear resolution left Stephens with mixed feelings. Bringing the radiation experiments to a halt was obviously a victory; no more patients would be harmed. Less satisfying was the mysterious, secretive way the studies were stopped. "I probably would have never written about the whole thing if it had been better known over the years," Stephens says. The researchers were never sanctioned, and no one told the research subjects or their families the truth about what had happened. The local press paid little attention. In December 1973, Saenger's research group received an award from the University of Texas for their work on total body irradiation. A junior member of the group, Edward Silberstein, sent Stephens a copy of the award announcement. He signed it, "Yours for bigger and better press conferences."[19]

· · ·

Most whistleblowers are victims of circumstance. They find themselves in trouble not of their own making that presents them with a hard moral choice: speak up or stay silent. Not Martha Stephens. She saw a fight brewing and she eagerly jumped into the fray. Today her social activism seems so natural that it's hard for me to imagine her any other way. She goes to rallies. She circulates petitions. She volunteers at women's shelters and soup kitchens. I've never seen her without a visor bearing some slogan related to peace and justice. "It is convenient, sometimes, to be a short person—almost everyone can read the message on my head," she wrote in her memoir. "Whenever I go around the town, people stop me to say, *I agree with your hat.*"[20] When I visited her in February of 2020, Stephens had decorated her visor to proclaim her support for Bernie Sanders. "When I wear my Bernie hat, people think my name is Bernie," she tells me.

Little in her upbringing would have predicted this particular future. Stephens grew up in a two-bedroom cottage in south Georgia in the 1940s and '50s, the oldest of three sisters. Like most small-town Southerners, her family went to church regularly, worshiping at the Disciples of Christ. Her father drove a soft drink delivery truck. When the United States joined the war and her father was drafted into the military, her mother started renting out one of their bedrooms to couples from a nearby air base. After the war, Martha's father became what she calls a "jobber" of general merchandise, calling on country stores in a van. Martha's mother, against the wishes of her husband, took a job as a legal secretary to help pay for Martha's tuition at the Georgia State College for Women. According to Martha, she was never especially engaged in politics back then. "I didn't do anything or get involved in much of anything," she says. "But what I always say is, 'I believed.' The beatitudes, I heard them in church, and I believed that you were supposed to help each other."

In 1961, Stephens was in graduate school at the University of Georgia, studying for a master's degree in English. "I was up in my carrel working on my thesis, just a little bookworm, a little wormy kind of person," she says. Feeling the need for some fresh air she went down from the upper floor to the front steps of the library. "Well, there was some kind of hoorah out on the walk in front of the library," she says. A crowd of people, mainly men, were chanting, "2-4-6-8, we don't want to integrate!" Coming down the walkway through the crowd was a group of three people, two of whom were guards. "In between these guards was a Black woman," Stephens says, hushing her voice almost to a whisper. "Charlayne Hunter-Gault." Hunter-Gault—who was named Charlayne Hunter at the time—was one of two African American students to integrate the University of Georgia that year. (Hamilton Holmes was the other one.)

"2-4-6-8, we don't want to integrate! I thought, What?" Students were lined up on either side of the walkway heckling Hunter. Seized by anger, Stephens stepped out onto the sidewalk, and as Hunter and the guards approached, she took Hunter's hand and said, "Charlayne, welcome to the university." At that moment, the cameras started to click. "Flashlights! Because the press was all there! Pictures!" Stephens shakes her head. "It's a wonder they let me do that. I don't know why they let me do that. I guess I looked like I couldn't possibly be a threat, this small woman."

"She's always been an activist," her husband, Jerone, says. "When we were in graduate school during the Vietnam War, it was just getting started and she and some of the other women in our complex took their babies in their strollers and began protesting around the complex." Jerone is a retired political scientist who spent most of his career at Bowling Green State University. He and Martha live apart now, although they still seem to spend a lot of time together. They have three grown children, two daughters and a son. Jerone and I are having lunch in February of 2020 at his favorite restaurant, a deli called Izzy's. "She's written hundreds of articles for the street paper, the poor people's paper," he says. "Every week she goes a couple of times to some protest. She's an influential voice in the city. Politicians listen to her when she opposes something."

Jerone and Martha met in the early 1960s in Clinch County,

Georgia, right on the edge of the Okefenokee Swamp, where they were both teaching school. Martha had finished her master's degree and was trying to save for a trip to Europe. Jerone, recently divorced, was planning to go to graduate school. He had moved to Clinch County to teach history, but he says that's not what qualified him for the job. "They said, 'Can you coach?' And I said, 'Yeah, I've been a coach.' And they said, 'Okay, you're hired.'" Jerone remembers standing outside the gym one day with a group of coaches when Martha came driving up in her Studebaker. "Betcha she hits the post," said one of the coaches. Martha hit the post.

Jerone is a tall, kindly man with a white beard and stray wisps of gray hair that fall over his ears. His voice seems so familiar that I keep wondering if we have met before, but eventually I decide that he just sounds like Will Geer. Jerone is a native Georgian, but unlike Martha, he grew up in the northern part of the state. His family ran a restaurant in Buford, a little town about 20 miles from the end of the Appalachian Trail. He says that going to Clinch County was like visiting a foreign country. "Being from North Georgia, anything below Atlanta was barbarian," he says. "It really was a wholly different culture. It really was, because it was the plantation." After he and Martha married, they moved to Paris, where Martha planned to study French at the Sorbonne, but they came back midway through the year when Martha got pregnant. Both finished their graduate work at the University of Indiana.

The longer Jerone and I talk, the more it sinks in how politically fraught it was to work as an American university professor in the 1960s. It seems as if every other name he or Martha mention is followed by the phrase "He lost his job" or "He was denied tenure." Jerone proudly informs me that he was fired from two jobs before winding up at Bowling Green State: first at Georgia State, his alma mater, and then at the University of Cincinnati. Both times it was about politics, especially his activism on civil rights and the war. At Cincinnati, Jerone was the faculty adviser to Students for a Democratic Society. "You couldn't be political during that time because the universities were still in favor of the Vietnam War," Jerone says. This was why he and a couple of young untenured colleagues formed the Junior Faculty Association. "We were opposed by the tenured faculty," Jerone says.

Jerone says he's surprised Martha never got fired. It probably helped that her department chair agreed with her about the radiation experiments. Later, some colleagues in her department tried to deny her tenure, Jerone tells me, but her academic record was too good. "They brought up things like the way she dressed," Jerone says. "How did she dress?" I ask. Jerone replies, "Mostly clothes from the Salvation Army." Then he starts to laugh. "It used to be a joke among our close friends that I was criticizing Martha for spending so much money on clothes."

For Jerone, the most disturbing thing about Saenger's radiation experiments was not the military funding (although that was obviously an issue) but the instrumental nature of the studies. "Here it was that they were irradiating people who were vulnerable people, who were working, and they were doing it in the way of clandestine movement," he says. "The Appalachians and the Blacks were always fearful of having to go to what was then called General Hospital, because they were treated as—what the doctors used to say—either 'research material' or 'clinical material.' That's the way they spoke of them. So that just hit a chord."

The first time I was in Cincinnati, Jerone gave me an article on research ethics he had published in the journal *Politics and Society* back in 1973.[21] I'll confess I didn't look at it right away. But once I sat down on my front porch and started to read, I could feel the back of my neck start to tingle. This was no ordinary academic paper. This was a prophecy. For Jerone, bureaucratic mechanisms such as consent forms, research guidelines, and IRBs are an elaborate ruse designed to hide the genuine issue in medical research, which is power. Doctors have it and their subjects don't. To claim that a signed consent form would protect powerless people was at best disingenuous and at worst an elaborate con job. "It is the exercise of power, not individual choice to submit to experimentation or overt societal authority, that is the core to understanding the whole process of human experimentation," he wrote.[22] "Until the issue is joined on the basis of power, rather than over smokescreens like ethical codes, exploitation will continue."[23]

And continue it has. The smoke screens have gotten thicker; the codes and regulations have grown ever more elaborate; and the methods of exploitation have evolved, like an exotic organism adapting to a new ecosystem. Today's system of protecting human subjects is a bureaucracy straight out of Kafka, a maze of commissions, consultants, compliance officers, accreditation bodies, professional societies, webinars, training courses, and for-profit ethics review boards, all devoted to research protection yet invisible to research subjects themselves. Virtually every major academic medical center employs a squad of functionaries whose primary directive is to shield the institution from sanctions and litigation. It feels like an elaborate betrayal. Jerone saw it all coming.

Later that evening, I have Singapore noodles with Martha and Jerone at the Blue Gibbon, a Chinese restaurant in Paddock Hills, where everyone seems to know Martha by name. In the parking lot afterward, as we stand by our cars in the dark, Martha says, "Well, it's no wonder it's so easy for us to talk to one another. We're all Southerners." We're saying our goodbyes when a cashier runs out of the restaurant waving my credit card, which I managed to leave on the table. From the Blue Gibbon I drive back to The Netherland Plaza, an elegant art deco hotel in downtown Cincinnati, where a jazz quartet is playing in the bar. The quartet is led by a trombonist playing standards in the old Tommy Dorsey style, coat and tie, balding with a distinguished gray goatee. It feels good to sit up front like Cole Porter with a double shot of Woodford Reserve, snowflakes gently falling outside, listening to "Misty" and thinking about treachery.

· · ·

On January 4, 1994, Martha Stephens was leaving home to teach her first class of the winter semester when she got a phone call from WKRC, a local television station. A copy of the 1972 Junior Faculty Association report had been dropped off at their newsroom, courtesy of an unknown informant. A recent discovery had prompted renewed interest in Saenger's experiments. Stephens made plans to talk to them the next day, but when she finished class that afternoon, she found a cameraman and a reporter waiting outside her office with a yellowing copy of the JFA report. Stephens had not seen the report in years. After reading it over she gave the reporters a blunt assessment on the record. "No consent form would have been valid for these experiments unless it had said, 'You may die of radiation sickness within forty days if you accept this treatment,'" Stephens said on camera. "And of course, no form said that—or there would not have been any subjects."[24]

Twenty-two years had passed since the initial controversy over Saenger's experiments. But on November 15, 1993, Eileen Welsome, an investigative journalist for the *Albuquerque Tribune*, had published the first installment of a three-part series called "The Plutonium Experiment."[25] Welsome had discovered that medical researchers working on behalf of the US military in the 1940s had secretly injected unwitting patients with plutonium to see how it traveled through the body. Welsome had identified the victims by name and tracked down their families in locations all over the country. The shock of her revelations jolted Cincinnati journalists into looking at the radiation experiments that they had ignored in 1972.

A few days after Stephens's appearance on WKRC, the station called again. They wanted her to discuss the radiation experiments on their Sunday morning news show, *Newsmakers*. The producer of *Newsmakers* hoped for a dramatic confrontation with a defender of the experiments, David Mann, a Harvard-educated attorney and a Democratic member of the US House of Representatives. The prospect filled Stephens with dread.[26] Jerone was on sabbatical in Central America. All their allies in the Junior Faculty Association had left the university. Her children had no memory of the events of 1972, and most of her activist friends knew nothing about them. Stephens didn't even watch television news shows. She had no idea whether *Newsmakers* would provide her with a fair forum.

Something else was bothering her. When Stephens was around thirteen years old, she was chosen to give a speech on stage for a school graduation ceremony. Toward the end of her speech, she looked down at her papers and found that she couldn't read them. The lights on the stage were making it impossible for her to see the words. She froze. "I mean, I couldn't finish. I couldn't say anything," Stephens tells me. Even more humiliating was the presence of a friend's grandmother laughing hysterically in the front row. "Oh, God. So, I probably cried and walked off the stage," Stephens says. "That will really mark you. Yeah, that kind of thing can mark you." It took decades for her to work up the courage to give another public talk. Even today Stephens gets upset if she sees an embarrassed child stumbling through a speech, especially a girl. "I have to go find them and say, 'You'll be okay. You did fine.'"

At first Stephens tried to weasel out of the appearance on *Newsmakers*. But eventually she worked up the courage to do it, and if the results were any indication, she did very well. Her opponent changed his mind. Soon Mann was calling for the victims to be compensated. Local reporters started to contact Stephens, who still had copies of the radiation study documents squirreled away in her basement. By the end of January, Nick Miller, of the *Cincinnati Post*—the city's afternoon newspaper—had published the first print story on the experiments. The front-page headline read, "The Secret History of UC's Radiation Tests."[27] To Stephens, it felt like a miracle.[28]

Like Eileen Welsome, Nick Miller had decided it was critical to include stories of the research subjects, even if there was little information to go on. He led with the story of Subject 022, a forty-eight-year-old woman with lung and spinal cancer who was later identified as Evelyn Jackson. When Saenger's team irradiated Jackson, she began to deteriorate. She vomited. She became weak. She started to hallucinate. Within ten days, Jackson was dead. Miller wrote, "She had no idea that as she suffered, researchers observed her agony, made careful notes, and wrote reports for eventual delivery to the Pentagon's Defense Atomic Support Agency."[29]

Local reporters had trouble finding physicians who would comment on Saenger's experiments. According to Stephens, not a single local doctor was willing to go on the record. The only willing commentator was a physician from out of town: David Egilman, an occupational health specialist at Brown University. Egilman had learned about Saenger's experiments in the 1980s when he was working as a medical officer in Cincinnati for the National Institute for Occupational Safety and Health. Egilman, along with Geoffrey Sea, a labor organizer, had tried for years to get reporters interested in Saenger's research without any real success. When the story resurfaced in 1994, Egilman was eager to join the fight. Not only did he speak to reporters; Egilman testified in two congressional hearings, telling a subcommittee that Saenger's research may have resulted in as many as twenty-two deaths.[30]

To Stephens, the obvious next move was finding the families of victims. She brought up this idea to reporters, but they couldn't convince their editors to devote any resources to the effort. One evening at home, Stephens was lamenting the problem with her friend, Laura Schneider, a graduate student in the Department of English. Stephens wondered if she could track down the families herself. The problem was her poor vision. She just didn't have the ability to pore over old records and microfilm. Schneider offered to do it for her, but Stephens refused, telling her she needed to work on her dissertation. To which Schneider replied, "But I don't *like* my dissertation. I'd rather do this."[31] As it turned out, Schneider had a knack for the job.

Schneider took the information from the study documents and started matching it up with funeral archives, obituaries, court bulletins, and other public records. Soon Schneider had found her first victim: Irene Shuff, a woman with lung cancer who had died twenty-four days after she was irradiated. Eventually, Schneider came up with a list of eighteen names. Stephens started calling the families, most of whom had no idea that a family member had ever been part of Saenger's experiments. Then she called Bob Newman, a human rights attorney, who filed a lawsuit on behalf of four surviving families.

In December 1993, the uproar over Eileen Welsome's series in the *Albuquerque Tribune* led Hazel O'Leary, the US Secretary of Energy, to launch an investigation into the government's secret radiation experiments. A month later O'Leary appointed bioethicist Ruth Faden, of Johns Hopkins University, to lead the investigation. The committee Faden directed, known as the Advisory Committee on Human Radiation Experiments (ACHRE), would eventually undertake the most wide-ranging investigation of a medical research scandal in US history. And once again, Stephens held her breath, hoping that justice would finally be served.

• • •

To Stephens, the reason she got involved in the radiation controversy should be obvious. "I live among people, writers, with a moral take on human life," she tells me. "Most of our great writers do have a vision of what life might be like." This is why she cared so much about the radiation experiments. "I mean, Vonnegut. John Milton. Charles Dickens, Faulkner to a large extent. I live with people with a moral view of life." She says some of her students would have preferred that she kept her moral opinions to herself. "We're trying to learn the structure of novels," they'd tell her. "We're not trying to learn peace and justice out of them." But many of them appreciated the moral message and remembered it long afterward. "All these writers I was teaching, they cared," Stephens says. "Why wouldn't I care?"

While I don't doubt Stephens's sincerity, I'm not sure her experience is generalizable. It hasn't been my experience that professors of literature are any more likely to care about wrongdoing than, say, professors of anthropology, political science, or history. Nor am I convinced that writing fiction is all that closely connected with a morally admirable life. Norman Mailer stabbed his wife in the stomach with a penknife. William S. Burroughs killed his wife with a gunshot to the head. Roald Dahl was an anti-Semite; J. D. Salinger was a sexual predator; Gertrude Stein collaborated with the fascist Vichy government in France. Even the sainted Dickens had a few skeletons in his closet.

It is true, of course, that fiction can deliver a powerful moral message. But moral zeal often transforms fiction writers into heavy-handed propagandists, clubbing the reader into submission with the force of their convictions. For every Charles Dickens there are hundreds of Ayn Rands. This may be why there are so few good novels about whistleblowing, a topic that does not easily lend itself to moral subtlety. Even the great John le Carré, a master at painting shades of gray in his Cold War novels of spycraft and political intrigue, lost all capacity for nuance when he turned to pharmaceutical industry wrongdoing. In *The Constant Gardener*, there are no moral dilemmas in blowing the whistle, no dueling loyalties, only light and darkness, heroes and villains.

In 1973, Stephens published her first book, *The Question of Flannery O'Connor*. O'Connor was a Catholic writer from southern Georgia who has never been accused of lacking a moral vision, even if the nature of that vision is missed by many readers. O'Connor captures the manners and language of backwoods Southerners with a comic precision that could easily come off as parody, but as Stephens points out, her vision of modern human life is as unremittingly dark as any work of literature this side of medieval Christendom. In O'Connor's fiction, nobody is safe. Sodom always brings down fire and brimstone. It's not the country primitives who suffer worst but the smug, self-satisfied men and women who feel certain they have risen above it all. A raging bull, a thieving Bible salesman, an escaped convict with a gun: disaster forces O'Connor's deluded characters to see themselves as they really are, sometimes only seconds before they meet a violent death. As Stephens writes, these disasters "are presented, typically, as blessings in disguise, really as acts of grace."[32]

O'Connor's short story "The Lame Shall Enter First" is told from the point of view of a well-intentioned, self-satisfied widower called Sheppard, who is a part-time counselor at a juvenile reformatory.[33] Sheppard is raising his ten-year-old son, Norton, by himself. Sheppard wants his son to be a good person, but Norton is a disappointment—a dim, selfish child who squirts ketchup on his cake and howls in grief for his dead mother. Sheppard feels certain his son is destined for a morally distasteful career as a banker, or even worse, the operator of a small loan company. If only Norton could understand that

children at the juvenile reformatory have it so much worse—
children such as Rufus Johnson, a fourteen-year-old boy with
a clubfoot who was forced to root around in garbage cans for
food. Yes, Rufus has a criminal history, but just look at all the
deprivations he has suffered. It would be so much different if
he had a father figure to model good behavior for him. Sheppard decides to bring Rufus into his house to live, as a moral
lesson for Norton.

Sheppard is relentlessly kind. He buys Rufus a telescope,
and then a microscope. He orders a specially designed shoe for
Rufus's clubfoot and delivers long lectures on science and psychology. But Rufus is a sneering demon who responds to kindness with gratuitous insults. He uses foul, racist language and
orders Norton around like a servant. When he discovers the
unused room of Norton's dead mother, he goes to her closet,
puts on her corset, and parades around the room like a vaude-
ville stripper. "Satan's got me in his power!" he snarls. When
Sheppard patiently explains that God is an invention designed
to comfort the ignorant, Rufus replies that Satan has Sheppard in his power too. "The dead are judged and the wicked
are damned. They weep and gnash their teeth while they burn
and it's everlasting darkness," Rufus says, adding, "Satan runs
it." At every turn Rufus rebels against his forced enrollment
in Sheppard's liberal reeducation camp. "God, kid, how do you
stand it?" he asks Norton. "He thinks he's Jesus Christ." Norton is enthralled. He is learning moral lessons, but they're not
the ones that Sheppard intended.

Sheppard's moment of clarity comes when Rufus is
arrested for vandalism and burglary. As Rufus is hauled away
by the police, he falsely accuses Sheppard of sexually molest-
ing him. Afterward, Sheppard sits in the dark telling himself, "I have nothing to reproach myself with. I did more for
him than I did for my own child." But as he repeats the words
silently, his face goes pale with self-revulsion. He really had

done more for Rufus than for his own child. "He had stuffed his own emptiness with good works like a glutton," O'Connor writes. Sheppard rushes upstairs to tell Norton that he loves him, but he is too late. He sees Norton's body hanging in a "jungle of shadows, just below the beam from which he had launched his flight into space."[34]

It's not a subtle story. I'm not even sure it's a good one. But the character of Sheppard is such a damning portrait of the insufferable, moralizing do-gooder that I can't help but wonder, "Is that how I appear to other people?" The thought is disturbingly plausible. I've heard the accusation before, and it stung. Maybe I'm just stuffing my emptiness with good works like a glutton, so certain of my position on the moral high ground that I lecture and patronize anyone who sees things differently. If I were a character in a Flannery O'Connor story, this would be my flash of insight, a moment of grace just before the bull rushes in to gore me to death on his horns.

When I raise this possibility to Stephens, she replies, "Well, you *and* me." But Stephens doesn't strike me as self-righteous, just fierce in her moral convictions. She says that many people can't believe that her long crusade on behalf of the radiation victims didn't come from some secret agenda. Yet there was no agenda, only moral principle. She had nothing to gain. Stephens is proud of what she did, and if she hadn't acted, she would have been ashamed of herself. "I would have felt real bad not to have wanted to blow the whistle on them," she says. She would have felt that way even if it had been riskier. "What chances have I taken in my life? I probably haven't taken many."

What is unusual about Martha Stephens is her deep, almost reflexive empathy for people in distress. Most of us would like to think we'd step out of a jeering crowd to welcome a solitary Black student to an all-white campus, but would we actually do it? I suspect Stephens would have done it even if she'd never picked up a novel by Vonnegut or Dickens. It is instinctive for her. Jerone says this is why Martha hates to spend money on clothes or in restaurants. "Every time she spends a dollar she thinks, 'A poor person could use that,'" Jerone says. "When she traveled with me in Latin America, she cried all the time. Because she'd see a poor person, and she just would break down crying. And in Latin America where I traveled, I saw *all* poor people."

Over the course of our conversations, I keep pressing Stephens on what moved her to get involved with this particular controversy—why, of all the righteous fights she might have picked, she chose this one. Sometimes she brings up the Vietnam War. "I'd been on marches in Washington about it. It was a horrible thing," she says. "And then this idea that there was this war research? I thought, 'Well, we'll stop this if we can.'" But more often our conversation turns to patients, especially the women. Stephens speaks about these women as if she knew them personally.

"Maude Jacobs, I'll never forget Maude Jacobs," Stephens says to me one afternoon in her kitchen. "She had small children, no husband. She had breast cancer. She got a call one day from the hospital and they said, 'We've got a new treatment for your cancer. Can you come over tomorrow and get it?' And so she did. Her daughter said she put on her hat and called a taxi and was picked up and taken to the hospital." Saenger gave Jacobs 150 rads of total body irradiation. She went back home that day, but she vomited all night. Her older daughter took her back to the hospital. She only lasted three weeks. "Well, Maude Jacobs never left that room," Stephens says. "She never saw her children again. They weren't allowed to visit. In those days you couldn't have children visit. And she died."

When I ask why Maude Jacobs had lodged so deeply in her memory, Stephens says, "I don't know. She was a pretty woman, just trying to take care of her kids. A Southerner, like I am. She was from Kentucky." Death came so quickly for Jacobs that she didn't even have time to make arrangements for her children. The younger ones were sent to an orphanage. "When her children at home learned that she had died, one of them ran away from home," Stephens says. "She couldn't hear any more about it. She couldn't hear any more about not seeing her mother again. She ran outside and spent the night in a culvert." The thought upsets Stephens even after all these years. "Who can hear that and not react to it?" she asks. "Who could hear those stories and just say, 'Oh well'? I don't get it."

• • •

In late 1993, when the Clinton administration announced the creation of the Advisory Committee on Human Radiation Experiments (ACHRE), American bioethicists saw it as a milestone event, a mark of legitimacy for a still-young academic field. ACHRE consisted of a fourteen-member advisory commission and fifty-six-member support staff. Yet the size of ACHRE was more than matched by the magnitude of the task it faced. The federal government had sponsored thousands of ionizing radiation experiments over a period of many decades, many of them on highly vulnerable populations. A federal directive had produced nearly six million pages of documents for the commission to review.[35] Over a period of eighteen months, the commission interviewed over nineteen hundred individuals and held public meetings all over the country. Its cost exceeded $6 million.[36]

Martha Stephens expected the worst. ACHRE included no research subjects or surviving family members. The public meetings were short on detail and long on philosophical abstraction, devoting hours to theoretical questions such as "What is informed consent?" When three members of the

committee came to Cincinnati in October 1994 for a public hearing, it seemed obvious to Stephens that they had not
studied or prepared. They had simply sat on their risers in a
hotel conference room, listening to members of eleven families speak.[37] Newspapers reported extended debates among
committee members about the perils of judging the misdeeds
of the past by current ethical standards. For people like Martha and Jerone Stephens, who had been outraged by Saenger's
experiments at the very time when they were taking place, an
argument about the difficulties of retrospective moral judgment sounded suspiciously like yet another cover-up.

On October 3, 1995, ACHRE released its final report in a
White House ceremony.[38] The conclusions were disappoint-
ing, although not as bad as Martha Stephens had feared. It was
true that the advisory committee didn't clearly recommend
that the families of the Cincinnati victims be financially compensated, as many family members had hoped.[39] It didn't even
give an unequivocal recommendation that they deserved an
apology. At times the committee appeared to bend over backward to avoid offense to the medical profession. But there was
enough condemnation of Saenger's experiments for Stephens
and the families to make a plausible declaration of victory,
even if it didn't quite feel that way.[40]

Not everyone was as forgiving of ACHRE as Stephens was.
"This report is the worst thing to happen to medical ethics
since the Bible," David Egilman said.[41] What upset Egilman
were the ethical contortions performed by the advisory committee to avoid assigning blame to the physicians and scientists whose actions they condemned.[42] ACHRE had also
decided that if an unwitting victim had not been harmed, it
was not necessary to notify that victim or their family that they
had been experimented upon. This made no sense to Egilman.
If your rights were violated, you deserve to know about it, full
stop. Egilman told me, "If you're raped, do you not get told you

were raped—if, say, you were drunk or given a roofie? Unless there's a vaginal tear or a rectal tear?"

According to Eileen Welsome, the families of victims were bitterly disappointed. "I guess the government really won. All the culprits that planned and executed this thing got away with it," said the nephew of one subject. Another man's mother was given a radioactive iron cocktail at Vanderbilt University when he was a fetus. He told Welsome, "I do feel betrayed and I feel abused by this committee's report."[43] Nor was there much sense of public vindication. By the time the ACHRE report came out, the public had stopped paying attention. Most Americans were far more interested in the verdict in O. J. Simpson's murder trial, which was announced on the same day.[44] The *New York Times* buried its story on the radiation report on page 19.

Yet the ACHRE report was not the last word on the case. The Cincinnati victims had launched a class-action lawsuit, *Shuff v. Saenger*, in 1994. It was a long, ugly fight that took five years to resolve. Each of the thirteen defendants from the University of Cincinnati hired their own counsel, mostly from high-powered Cincinnati law firms. Also taking part were legal representatives for the Department of Justice, the Defense Nuclear Agency, the city of Cincinnati, and the University of Cincinnati. At times there were as many as twenty-eight attorneys in the courtroom. When the case was finally settled in May of 1999, it was for a sum of $5.4 million.[45] Most families got about $50,000.[46] Just having the lawsuit finished was a relief. After five years of legal maneuvering, bitter arguments, and agonizing revelations of medical harm, many family members were simply exhausted.

In the end, the most rancorous point of contention was not money, but honor. Family members wanted an apology from Eugene Saenger, the architect of the study. Saenger refused, telling the families through his attorney that an apology was "nonnegotiable." As a concession, the defendants proposed a small, 12-by-25-inch plaque at the hospital inscribed with the words "In Memoriam," along with the initials of the victims. Negotiations finally produced the small plaque I saw hidden in the shrubbery. Some families held a commemorative service at the hospital, but others found the memorial so objectionable they refused even to visit.[47]

. . .

How do you repair the wrongs of an unethical experiment? The Cincinnati researchers deceived their patients, shortened their lives, and subjected them to agonizing deaths, yet the wrongs of the experiment go beyond physical harm. A deep wound also comes from being used as what Jerone Stephens called "research material." To be treated as "material" was a humiliation, an injury to their self-respect. What their families needed was a way for their honor to be restored. An honest memorial might have helped, but the simplest way to restore a person's injured self-respect is to apologize.

An apology, according to psychiatrist Aaron Lazare, is an "exchange of humiliation and power."[48] The humiliation to research subjects comes from being treated as objects. Not only do many subjects feel degraded by their treatment, but they also feel ashamed they have allowed it to happen. They may feel that they should have known better, that they failed to protect themselves, that they allowed themselves to be conned, bullied, or deceived. An apology reverses this by transferring the humiliation back to the researchers. The researchers become the ones who are unethical or incompetent, while the victims are given power. Their power comes from the ability to extend or withhold forgiveness.

This reversal is precisely why so many researchers refuse to apologize. To repair the injured honor of a victim demands a blow to your own. To apologize is to lower yourself, not just in the eyes of others but in your own eyes. You must acknowledge your own failures, weaknesses, or mistakes. For most researchers, this is simply a step too far. I suspect this is why Eugene Saenger refused to apologize and why administrators at the University of Cincinnati have given their memorial plaque such shabby treatment over the years. To honor the victims properly would require an honest appraisal of their own sins.

Apologies to research subjects are rare, but when they are offered, they usually come in the form of a public statement. Public apologies differ from private apologies in important ways. A private apology can be fumbling, awkward, and emotional. It can even be improvised on the fly. But the words must be heartfelt and sincere. Public apologies, in contrast, don't require much sincerity to do their work. Public apologies are spoken for posterity. Their purpose is to restore the dignity of the victims for the public record. For this reason, public apologies tend to be carefully scripted documents prepared in advance and delivered in ritualized fashion.[49]

It is easy to ruin an apology. Some people phrase their apologies in a way that makes the situation worse. To say, "I'm sorry you were offended," for example, is a pseudo-apology that casts blame on the victim. Apologies can also be vague, defensive, or conditional: "If anyone was harmed or inconvenienced, I apologize." The grand master of bad apologies was Richard Nixon, whose famous "Checkers" speech in 1952 was a cheesy, self-serving justification for bad behavior masquerading as a mea culpa. Twenty-two years later, when Nixon was forced to resign the presidency, he could have exited with a sincere apology. Instead, he tried to justify his crimes. Nixon said, "I would say only that if some of my judgments were wrong, and some were wrong, they were made in what I believed at the time to be the best interests of the nation."[50]

In his 1971 book, *Relations in Public*, the sociologist Erving

Goffman explained what an effective apology needed to do. Goffman, who could sound like an extraterrestrial observing the strange inhabitants of planet Earth, described the essential elements in clinically precise detail: an expression of chagrin, a repudiation of the offending action, the performance of penance, and the volunteering of restitution.[51] Penance and restitution are important partly because of the victim's need to see that the offender has suffered. But they also serve as a sign that an apology is sincere. An apology with no offer of restitution can easily come off as an empty gesture, like a restaurant owner who apologizes for poor service and cold food but refuses to offer the diner a refund.[52]

To his credit, President Clinton offered a sincere public apology to the victims of the government's human radiation experiments. He ignored the advice of ACHRE, which recommended apologies only to a small subset of victims, and he apologized not only to every victim but also to their families and their communities. Many of the radiation experiments, Clinton said, were "unethical not only by today's standards but by the standards of the time. They failed both the test of our national values and the test of humanity."[53] Yet the apology was not accompanied by restitution. Only a small fraction of the victims of human radiation experiments ever received financial compensation for the way they were mistreated.

Even rarer than apologies are memorials to victims of research abuse. Like apologies, memorials serve a moral purpose. What is disorienting about an inadequate social response to wrongdoing is how it disrupts our sense of the way the moral universe works. It is disconcerting to see innocent victims forgotten while transgressors are rewarded. This is why so many of us are disturbed by monuments to the great racist villains of history, such as Pitchfork Ben Tillman or Nathan Bedford Forrest. We would like to imagine that we live in a society that

reflects our sense of justice. Memorials, if constructed properly, can help ratify that moral vision.

Very few memorials honor the victims of research abuses.
The subjects in the Tuskegee syphilis experiment are exceptional in having two memorials: the Tuskegee History Center, a regional museum in Tuskegee that places the Tuskegee
experiment in the history of the civil rights movement, and
the Legacy Museum, which is located on the campus of Tuskegee University. The subjects of the Willowbrook hepatitis experiments don't have a memorial, but there is a marker
titled "Informed Consent" on the Willowbrook Mile, a walking trail on Staten Island that commemorates the role of the
Willowbrook State School in the cause of disability rights.

It was partly because such memorials are so rare that I
wanted to see the one commemorating the Cincinnati victims. When I showed my photos of the shabby, shrub-covered
plaque to Martha Stephens, she was not surprised. It was no
more than she expected of her university. After my visit, however, I posted a photo of the plaque on social media along with
the caption "How the University of Cincinnati buries its sins."
The story was picked up by a local television station, and the
resulting publicity forced the medical center to issue a statement. The medical center did not apologize, of course. But it
did say that the neglect was unintentional. When notified that
the memorial had been covered by bushes, the medical center
claimed that the issue was "addressed with new landscaping
within hours to prevent this from occurring again."[54]

. . .

It's a clear June afternoon in 2018, and once again I am standing in front of the plaque. This time I've come with Martha
Stephens and her old friend from the English department,
Dave Logan. The plaque is much easier to see now. Landscap-
ers have cleared away the shrubbery and replaced it with a

small bed of red and white flowers. They look freshly planted. The first thing Stephens does when she sees the plaque is to start identifying the victims. "The second one here, Margaret Bacon? She was the shortest survivor of all," Stephens says. "She lived six days." Logan wonders why the plaque lists only seventy victims. "It says 'presented by their families,'" he says, "but it was paid for by the lawsuit." I note that there is nothing on the plaque to let anyone know that these were research subjects. Stephens agrees. "You don't know a damn thing and it's facing the wrong way," she says.

Afterward, we wander inside to the Saenger Laboratory. Stephens asks staff members about the building where patients were irradiated. "The Frankenstein room!" says one man, who says he started working at the hospital in the 1980s. "The Frankenstein room?" I ask. "That's what we used to call it," he says, laughing. "If you were to see the room and everything, it looked like sci-fi. Big old table, big old equipment with arms and everything," he says. "It looked like they were making a Frankenstein monster." Stephens seems quite interested in this story. She says that this helps explain why the patients were so terrified.

A technician offers to show us the Saenger display. I'm not sure she has understood quite yet why we're here. "What's the big balloon glass thing?" Logan asks, pointing through the display case window. We speculate that it must have come from inside a piece of radiation equipment. Stephens is as polite as ever, but she seems intent on making certain that the technician understands how terrible Saenger's radiation experiments were. She asks the technician if she has ever heard about the experiments, but the technician dodges the question. Stephens says that she saw Saenger in court after the experiment came to light. "These two were involved in exposing it in 1972," I say, gesturing at Stephens and Logan. "That's why I'm here to talk to them." "Interesting!" the technician replies.

The technician is friendly and courteous, but she clearly doesn't seem comfortable acknowledging the horrors of what happened. It is possible she doesn't know the full story. Stephens tells her that Saenger's abuses made the University of Cincinnati famous and that she wrote a book about it called *The Treatment.* Many of the subjects in his studies died horrible deaths. "Hmm!" says the technician. After a while, we decide it's time to go. I feel a little relieved to be leaving. The conversation has turned awkward. As we say our goodbyes, Logan tells the technician, "It would be nice to put a copy of *The Treatment* in the display case, but I don't think that's going to happen." The technician agrees. She laughs politely as we exit.

CHAPTER 6

The Unfortunate Experiment

I t's a late spring evening at the Fisher House in Auckland, and I'm feeling a little awkward. I've been invited to a meeting of the Churchill Dining Club, a local historical society devoted to the veneration of Sir Winston Churchill. My host is Ron Jones, a retired obstetrician-gynecologist and one of three physicians who, many decades ago, blew the whistle on New Zealand's most notorious research scandal. I neglected to pack for the occasion, so I'm wearing a frayed blue jacket and a borrowed Knox College necktie that Jones has kept from his university days in the 1950s at the University of Otago.

The Fisher House is located in a homestead built by the manufacturing magnate Sir Woolf Fisher on his thoroughbred stud farm in the early 1960s. Horse portraiture lines the walls. After drinks at the bar, where I get a warm welcome from the group, Jones and I move to the former billiard room for dinner with a couple dozen club members, mostly men of a certain age. Their faces look as if they've been transported from a different era: a ruddy-faced gentleman with a handlebar mustache, a scarecrow wearing glasses. Next to me sits a retired pediatric radiologist who trained in Boston during the Watergate era. He cheerfully informs me that he plans to get up at 3 a.m. to watch the Trump impeachment hearings. Perched on an easel at the front of the dining room is a portrait of Sir Winston himself.

The meeting proceeds in what I understand to be the usual manner. After a generous plate of pork loin and potatoes, there is a trivia quiz about the life and accomplishments of Winston Churchill. (I score 0 for 20.) There are formal greetings from the Churchill Aficionados, a sister group in America, and a package of memorabilia for distribution. There are a number of speeches and readings, most of them less than two minutes long and timed by a dining club member with a stopwatch. For reasons I don't quite understand, the Swedish consul is in attendance. He stands and sings an a cappella rendition of "How Great Thou Art" in Māori. Ron Jones, my host, delivers a short talk about Churchill's school days at Harrow. "It is well known that Churchill was a dunce," Jones tells the group, with just a hint of a twinkle in his eye.

If there were an encyclopedia entry for "Kiwi gentleman," the accompanying photo would probably look something like Jones. At age eighty he is fit, tall, and brimming with good cheer. His manner is relaxed and unfailingly polite. When he's not wearing a jacket, he favors Hawaiian shirts and a floppy hat. Like many New Zealanders, he jokes easily with strangers, and his humor is gently self-deprecating. A few days earlier, we passed a couple of young people selling T-shirts. "People tell me I shouldn't wear those because of my turkey neck," Jones told them. "When people say things like that, you need to take their advice seriously." At a craft brewery, he gestured toward me and told the bartender, "He's never been here before, so he'll need to sample all thirteen beers." Jones grew up in a working-class family in Christchurch, on New Zealand's South Island, where his father worked in a slaughterhouse. He went to medical school at the University of Otago in Dunedin, about 220 miles south of Christchurch, and lived at Knox College, a residential college established by the Presbyterian Church. He says his time at Knox was life-changing, not least because of the expectations of the students. "We were gentlemen, and we were treated like gentlemen," he says. The motto of Knox College is *Gratia et Veritas*, or Grace and Truth.

Over thirty years ago, along with fellow physicians Bill McIndoe and Jock McLean, Jones helped expose the research scandal that New Zealanders call, with characteristic understatement, "the unfortunate experiment." Beginning in 1966, at National Women's Hospital, in Auckland, women with a precursor of cervical cancer—cervical cancer in situ, or CIS—were deceived and left untreated for decades. Many of them died. Jones, McIndoe, and McLean attempted for years to stop the experiment, but the public did not become aware of it until June 1987, when *Metro* magazine published an investigative report triggered by a scientific article the three physicians published in *Obstetrics and Gynecology*.[1] The shocking report in *Metro* led to a judicial inquiry, seven months of public hearings, and far-reaching governmental reforms. In the decades since Jones helped expose the unfortunate experiment, he has become the primary guardian of its legacy, mainly out of his Presbyterian sense of duty. "I wouldn't have had a clear conscience had I run away from this," he says.

Outside of New Zealand, few people have heard of the unfortunate experiment. It is rarely studied or taught, even in the field of bioethics, where scandals such as the Tuskegee syphilis study and the Willowbrook hepatitis study are a standard part of the curriculum. This is an odd oversight, and not just because of the severity of the ethical violations. It is one of the rare scandals where some measure of justice was eventually achieved. The victims were given a public forum, and the architect of the study, Herb Green, was forced to answer for it. Only his advanced age and poor health prevented Green from being sanctioned.

If not for the actions of Ron Jones, there is a good chance the unfortunate experiment would have never been exposed. Yet Jones seems haunted by his choice. It is only when he talks about the unfortunate experiment that his buoyant optimism gives way to despondency. "I've had a sense of guilt that without me, that terrible, terrible episode would never have happened," he says. "It's never out of my mind. There's not an hour of the day when some aspect of it raises its head in my life. And this is forty years later. I cannot escape it."

• • •

Academic physicians are not known for their modesty, but even among his peers George Herbert "Herb" Green stood out. Colleagues describe him as a bully. "Green was loud, big and aggressive," says the cytologist Michael Churchouse, who worked with Green for years. Conservative in his politics and belligerent in his personal style, Green was an obstetrician-gynecologist who opposed abortion and resisted sterilization. He once described cervical cancer screening (Pap smears) as "the biggest hoax ever perpetrated on women."[2] Green took pride in being seen as a contrarian—a "doubting Thomas," as he put it. His ability to intimidate others came partly from his size and bearing; Green was a large, gruff man who had grown up in gum boots on a south Otago farm. But his physical size was exceeded by his high self-regard. Green was supremely confident in his own judgment, and he was not shy about letting others know it. If egos were cars, Green's would have been a Cadillac Eldorado.

In the end, he drove it over a cliff. In New Zealand, Green is known as the physician behind the unfortunate experiment.

His tragic flaw was signaled by an Ogden Nash quote written on his office chalkboard: "Don't confuse me with the facts—my mind is made up."[3] Green was convinced that cervical carcinoma in situ (CIS)—a condition in which abnormal cells are found on the surface of the cervix but not yet any deeper—would not progress to invasive cervical cancer. Never mind the scientific evidence, or expert consensus, or even the policy at his hospital, all of which instructed that CIS should be treated by excision, not simply left alone. Green's confidence in his own judgment was unshakable. In 1966, with the approval of his hospital superiors, Green set out to prove his theory to the world, allowing his patients with CIS to go untreated for years without their knowledge or consent. At the time, only one of his colleagues opposed him.

At first glance, Bill McIndoe might have seemed a poor match for Green. He was quiet and small in stature. Unlike Green, he did not have a university appointment. A devout Presbyterian, McIndoe served as clerk of the session at his church in Epsom, a neighborhood in Auckland, where he sang in the choir and led a Bible class for twenty years. As a young man he had taken a pledge never to drink alcohol; at parties, he always drank orange juice. Friends and family members describe McIndoe as a gentle, self-effacing man with a generous sense of humor and a warm bedside manner. He called his patients "Sunshine." Yet McIndoe could be hardheaded. Once he dug his teeth into a problem, he refused to let it go.

McIndoe had come to medicine late. Raised by working-class Scots immigrants, he had originally trained as an electrician. He earned a BSc in physics by studying part-time at Auckland University. When World War II broke out, McIndoe worked in the radar division of the Department of Scientific and Industrial Research before transferring to the army. He married his wife, Noeline, on his final military leave. When the war ended, McIndoe set out on a new career, studying medicine at Otago Medical School. He had hoped to become a medical missionary for the Presbyterian Church, but that ambition was derailed by the birth of his first daughter. For several years McIndoe worked as a general practitioner in Hawera, a small town on the North Island, before he decided to start over yet again at National Women's Hospital, where, at the age of forty, he began specialty training in obstetrics and gynecology. He would eventually become the hospital's colposcopist.[4]

The colposcope is a diagnostic instrument used for pelvic exams. It looks like a set of World War II naval binoculars, but it functions like a microscope, allowing the clinician to look at a magnified view of the vagina, vulva, and cervix. Developed in Germany in the 1920s, the colposcope was originally used to detect cancers invisible to the naked eye. When Pap smears became a standard screening tool for cervical cancer, clinicians began using the colposcope to follow up on abnormal smears in order to define the lesion and take a diagnostic biopsy. National Women's Hospital had bought a colposcope in 1960, but the instrument had mostly gone unused until McIndoe discovered it in one of the operating theaters.[5] An amateur photographer who had used range finders in the military, McIndoe took up the colposcope with enthusiasm. For a time, he was the only colposcopist in the country.[6]

National Women's Hospital was founded in 1946. Within two decades, it had become New Zealand's most respected institution for women's health. Originally located in a military complex used by the American military to take care of service members but abandoned after the war, National Women's was moved in 1964 to a new building at the foot of Maungakiekie/One Tree Hill, a volcanic peak that is one of Auckland's best-known landmarks.[7] National Women's was officially closed in 2004, but the buildings are still intact. Prominently displayed on the grounds is a neoclassical marble statue of a shapely, half-draped woman with a plaque reading "Spirit of Peace."

It was no secret at National Women's that Herb Green held unorthodox views about CIS. Those views had evolved out of an understandable concern that women with CIS were being overtreated with hysterectomies. Green did not want to do anything that would unnecessarily cost young women their ability to bear children. But his concern about overtreatment had gradually hardened into a belief that CIS would not progress to invasive cancer. For years he had been taking a wait-and-see approach to the condition, even as evidence mounted that such an approach could be dangerous.[8]

On June 20, 1966, Green approached his colleagues with a plan to study the results of his approach formally.[9] The occasion was a staff meeting. When Bill McIndoe saw the agenda, he was alarmed. Not only had he not been consulted about the study—a study about which he had grave doubts—but he was expected to be personally involved. He was the study colposcopist. Only four days earlier, on June 16, Henry Beecher had published his famous article, "Ethics and Clinical Research," in the *New England Journal of Medicine*, warning of the dangers of unethical human experimentation.[10] But it is unlikely that the journal would have reached Auckland by June 20, and there is no indication that the staff of National Women's paid any attention to the article later.

Presiding over the staff meeting was Alger Warren, the medical superintendent. Also present was another important figure: Dennis Bonham, the head of the Postgraduate School of Obstetrics and Gynecology. Bonham was an Englishman who had established an academic reputation by taking part in an important perinatal mortality study in Britain. Unlike Green, Bonham had liberal political views and championed women in medicine. But his management style was fierce and autocratic. A product of the savagely competitive British medical system, Bonham had a bombastic manner that intimidated many staff members.[11] "The girls always used to be a little scared of coming up with him in the lift," Churchouse says. In his book, *Doctors in Denial,* Ron Jones remembers the very first time he caught a glimpse of Bonham. He had heard a loud voice in the next corridor. "The owner of the voice was a large man in a fresh white coat, wisps of dark, Brylcreemed hair combed over his bald pate. Not only was he shouting, he was also progressively dismembering a set of patient records, sending sheets of paper flying in his wake."[12]

When the staff meeting commenced, Green said nothing to alleviate McIndoe's concerns. His aim was "to prove that carcinoma in situ is not a premalignant disease," he told the group.[13] To demonstrate this, Green planned to study women under the age of thirty-five with carcinoma in situ, as confirmed by a limited biopsy. If the cervix looked normal to the naked eye and the patient had no clinical signs of cancer, Green would give the patient "no further treatment." Instead, he would follow up with regular examinations and treat the patient only if the lesion progressed to invasive cancer.

McIndoe's alarm at Green's plan was understandable. Invasive cervical cancer is a deadly disease. During the first half of the twentieth century, before the widespread adoption of cervical screening, it was one of the leading causes of cancer-related deaths among women. By 1966, the evidence that CIS could progress to invasive cervical cancer had been mounting for decades.[14] According to Neville Hacker, a past president of the International Gynecologic Cancer Society, by the time Green approached his colleagues with the study in 1966, "there was almost universal agreement that CIS was a premalignant lesion."[15] Green's proposal even violated hospital policy, which stated that CIS should be treated with cone biopsy.[16] In a cone biopsy, or conization, the physician removes the abnormal cells by cutting out a small, cone-shaped wedge of tissue around them. Today conization is a relatively simple outpatient procedure, but even in the 1960s, conization carried few serious risks other than a small effect on a woman's ability to bear children and increased risk of preterm births for women who became pregnant.

Green had paid little attention to the design of his study. In fact, the study scarcely had much of a design at all. It had no control group against which the treatment of his subjects could be compared. Nor did it have any stopping rules— the guidelines for terminating a study if subjects are being harmed or disadvantaged. It had no Data and Safety Monitoring Board (DSMB) and no provisions for informed consent. For the women under Green's care, there was a lot to lose and little to gain apart from being spared the discomfort of conization.

When the staff meeting commenced, McIndoe spoke out to his colleagues. "I can hear his voice in my head. He would be spelling it out slowly and carefully," Mary Whaley, his daughter, says. But speaking out made no difference. Neither did a written memorandum.[17] In fact, an objection by the lowly McIndoe apparently counted for so little that most of his colleagues didn't even remember it later. As Whaley said later, "On one side were the people who made all the noise and did all the shouting, and on the other side was this shy little man in the corner saying he thought Green was wrong."[18] The senior staff approved Green's proposal over McIndoe's objections and passed it up the ladder to the Hospital Medical Committee, which approved it unanimously.

From 1966 onward, National Women's had two parallel treatment tracks for women with cervical carcinoma in situ, according to Ron Jones.[19] The first track consisted mainly of private patients managed by members of the "visiting" staff— the practitioners who did not have academic appointments. Those women got standard treatment. The second track consisted mainly of women at the public clinic, who were directed to Green. Those women got Green's "conservative" approach, which meant that Green monitored their CIS but did not remove the lesion.

From the very start, Green was confident that these women would be fine. He was convinced that CIS had nothing to do with cervical cancer. On the day his proposal was accepted in 1966, the minutes of the staff meeting state that women with CIS should be passed on to Professor Green, *"whose conscience is clear* and who could therefore accept complete responsibility for whatever happens" (italics added).[20]

• • •

When the research scandals of the past are remembered, the events unfold in a fixed direction, as if guided by the Presbyterian doctrine of predestination. Success or failure, salvation or damnation: everything is foreordained according to God's will. But at the time when events are taking place, nothing about them feels predestined. They don't even seem predictable. The narrative is halting and uncertain. It is filled with blind alleys, makeshift tactics, and failed plans. Nobody can figure out how the story will end or who will prevail. The characters don't know the plot, because there's no script. There's just improvisation.

After Green's study began in 1966, McIndoe improvised. His conscience bothered him, but he continued to provide colposcopic services for Green. The two men even managed to work together in relative peace for a while. But eventually, McIndoe grew more concerned. He was uncomfortable with his role in the study. He began pressing Green to bring his patients into the hospital for surgery. Their arguments could last for hours. But McIndoe never convinced Green to change his mind. "I can only assume," McIndoe later wrote, "that I have never been sufficiently belligerent and offensive for my comments and concern to be noted."[21]

In September 1973, McIndoe got his second wind. National

Women's was hosting a distinguished international visitor: Per Kolstad, the head of gynecological cancer at the Norwegian Radium Hospital and an expert in colposcopy. McIndoe asked him for an outside opinion about Green. After examining six of Green's patients and discussing six more, Kolstad made it clear not just that he believed CIS should be treated, but that Green's patients had been badly neglected.[22]

By this point, McIndoe had found a welcome ally in the hospital. Jock McLean was a pathologist, not an obstetrician-gynecologist; he spent his workday looking at tissue through a microscope. McLean could see direct evidence of how Green's patients were faring, and he did not like what he saw. One of his primary responsibilities was to evaluate the cone biopsy slides that came from the histology section of the laboratory. McLean had grown alarmed at how CIS lesions gradually progressed beyond the cervix to the vagina, vulva, and beyond—a progression he called "the creeping kiss."[23]

McLean had been appointed the charge pathologist at National Women's in 1961. Like McIndoe, he had grown up in a working-class family in Auckland and served in the army before attending Otago Medical School. In most ways, though, he and McIndoe couldn't have been more different. McLean was tall and carried himself with a military bearing. He saw the hospital establishment figures as stuffed shirts and preferred to socialize with the laboratory staff. "Good old Jock," says Churchouse, the cytologist. "He was a bit of a mad guy, a good guy, but eccentric. I liked him because he called a spade a spade." An unpretentious man who played up his own eccentricity, McLean drove a green Scimitar sports car and wore tweed jackets with elbow patches. His desk was overflowing with papers, journals, and boxes of glass pathology slides. He enjoyed a drink, flirted with women, and liked to have a good time. "Scratch my surface and you'll find the real me underneath," he often said.[24]

In October of 1973, spurred by Kolstad's September visit, McIndoe and McLean took action. It was the sort of action expected of sober-minded professionals intent on playing by the rules: reasoned memoranda submitted respectfully to hospital authorities. McIndoe prepared a twelve-page document with a list of seven women who had developed cancer under Green's policy.[25] McLean's memorandum included a list of thirteen women whose cancer diagnoses had been delayed by inadequate early biopsies.[26] But their efforts were no match for the stonewalling mechanisms that bureaucracies typically use to quell dissent. The superintendent of the Auckland Hospital Board declined to act, tossing the complaints back to the hospital. Years passed before a hospital subcommittee was appointed to investigate, and when the subcommittee finally reached a decision, it merely admonished everyone involved for allowing personality differences to develop into conflicts.[27]

Burdened by a sense of complicity, McIndoe stopped providing Green with colposcopic services. Green simply continued without him. McIndoe grew despondent. He was forced to take stress leave from his job. Alternately agitated and depressed, he spent evenings alone in his study or the hospital trying to write.[28] McIndoe was not built for confrontation. Quarrels and personal friction upset him. "He hated conflict," says Mary Whaley. "And in fact, actually, you know, he really didn't allow anger in the house at all. We had to suppress those sorts of things." His wife, Noeline, recalled a car trip from Auckland to Wellington in the early 1980s in which McIndoe talked about the study for nine consecutive hours. "He was away every Sunday going through the records," she said. "He never stopped reading and writing. It totally took over his life."[29]

As a stubborn, principled Presbyterian, McIndoe simply could not find it in himself to give up. But neither could he see a way forward. Going to the press was not an option; McIndoe felt that this would destroy his credibility. He was frozen in place, paralyzed by his own sense of honor, and he probably would have remained there if not for a push by Ron Jones, a younger but no less principled man who shared his Presbyterian values.

• • •

For nearly a century, most roads to a medical career in New Zealand ran through Dunedin. Settled by Scottish Presbyterians in the mid-nineteenth century, Dunedin is home to the University of Otago, the country's oldest university and for many years the only place in the country to get a medical education. Nearly everyone involved in the controversy over the unfortunate experiment passed through Dunedin at some point, from McIndoe, McLean, and Jones to Herb Green himself. Judge Silvia Cartwright, who headed the judicial inquiry into the scandal, grew up in Dunedin and graduated from the University of Otago's Faculty of Law. Even the phrase "the unfortunate experiment" owes its provenance to Dunedin. It was coined by David Skegg, a leading critic of Green's study and the chair of the University of Otago's Department of Preventive and Social Medicine.[30] The unfortunate experiment may have taken place in Auckland, but Dunedin is the city where its genealogy began and ended.

I moved to Dunedin with Ina in 1990, two years after the Cartwright Report was released and two weeks after our wedding. I had won a postdoctoral fellowship at the University of Otago's newly established Bioethics Research Centre, where I planned to work with Grant Gillett, a Kiwi neurosurgeon with a doctorate in philosophy from Oxford. We arrived on a rainy winter night in August and took a taxi from the airport to a granny flat on London Street, just up from the Albert Arms pub and a short walk away from Knox Church. We had booked the flat by mail from a retired police officer, no deposit required.

Thirty years ago, a trip from America to Dunedin felt like a journey to the end of the world. Part of the reason was geographical. Located on the southeastern coast of New Zealand's South Island, Dunedin is one of the more remote regions of an island nation that still felt like a far-flung outpost of the British Empire. But there was more to it than geography. It felt as if we had stepped into a time machine and emerged decades earlier. Small children wore hand-knitted sweaters. Milk was delivered to our door in bottles. The house we eventually rented came with a rotary push mower for the lawn and a hand wringer for wet laundry. The steep, twisting roads of Dunedin were filled with British vehicles from another era: Morris Minors from the 1940s, Mini Coopers from the 1960s and '70s. Ina and I paid $400 for a 1974 Hillman Hunter, mustard yellow and shaped like a shoebox. It looked as if it had been hand drawn by a first grader.

I knew nothing about the unfortunate experiment before I arrived in Dunedin, but learning about it didn't take long. It was already part of the medical curriculum. The new director of the Bioethics Research Centre, Alastair Campbell, had subjected Green's study to harsh criticism in his testimony to the Cartwright Inquiry, as had David Skegg. Even more deeply involved was Charlotte Paul, a University of Otago epidemiologist who had served as one of the Inquiry's three medical advisers. Nobody I met defended Green's study. Kiwis take a justifiable measure of pride in their long tradition of progressive politics; New Zealand was the first self-governing country in the world to give women the right to vote. The fact that the unfortunate experiment had exploited vulnerable women felt like a stain on the national honor.

We settled into Dunedin easily. To me, a lapsed Presbyterian who had once lived in Scotland, everything about the city looked familiar and just a little sideways, as if maybe I had dreamed it once. The streets had Scottish names lifted from Edinburgh and Glasgow: George, Princes, Argyle, Moray. A statue of Robert Burns stood on a pedestal in the center of town, usually with a seagull perched on his head. A church, a street, and a college all bore the name of John Knox. The university was a dead ringer for Glasgow University, where I did my doctorate in philosophy, and the Albert Arms, where Ina and I soon became regulars, was decorated in tartan plaid. Even the name Dunedin turned out to be the Gaelic word for Edinburgh.

Yet the Pacific air in Dunedin was like nothing I had smelled before, so clean and thin that it was like inhaling pure oxygen. It was as if the Presbyterian gloom of the Scots had been aired out and expanded, the dour fatalism leavened by smiles and open arms. It didn't hurt that the physical location was stunning. Dunedin sits among steep hills overlooking a harbor, on the other side of which lies the rugged Otago Peninsula. The setting looks like a cross between the lush green landscape of Ireland, the white beaches of Fiji, and the soaring cliffs of the Northern California coast. The town itself seemed remarkably egalitarian, devoid of great wealth or extreme poverty. If there were rich people in Dunedin, it was hard to tell where they lived.

Even more striking were the morals and manners of Dunedin. They were almost as old-fashioned as the cars. Shortly after we arrived, Ina and I got an invitation to dinner from the assistant master of Knox College, the residential college where Ron Jones had been taught how to behave as a gentleman. Coat and tie were expected. We ate with the Knox College staff and faculty members at "high table"—which, before that night, I had never realized was a literal description. The table was elevated, like a throne, so that we gazed out like lords over the dining hall, with the students sitting below us. Back home this would have felt absurd and uncomfortable. In Dunedin it just seemed anachronistic and charming, like my visit to the Churchill Dining Club.

Partly this was because everyone was so genuine and unguarded. People in Dunedin appeared immune to the jaded crust of cynicism that most Americans unconsciously adopt somewhere around the fifth grade. It wasn't simply that they were suspiciously kind, even to strangers. It was that they assumed the best of everyone. Sometimes I wondered if the entire region were governed by some kind of unspoken honor code. Bicycles stood unlocked. Fruit and vegetables sat unattended at roadside markets, with only an honor box nearby; the same was true for the *Otago Daily Times* in the Dunedin Public Hospital. Nearly twenty-five years later, I can remember walking across the campus of the University of Otago with my son, Crawford, and Nick Haslam, a family friend, who pointed to at least a dozen laptops spread out under trees and across the lawn. Nobody worried that they would be stolen.

The city wasn't without a dark side. Student life at the university had a rowdy, alcohol-driven culture that seemed hard to square with its scholarly image. And while safety didn't usually seem like a concern, only a few months after we arrived a mass shooting took place in the tiny settlement of Aramoana, only about 15 miles up the coast from Dunedin. Until the Christchurch mosque shootings in 2019, the Aramoana massacre was the deadliest mass shooting in New Zealand history. What seemed unusual about Dunedin was not any lack of tragedy or misfortune, but the calm, pragmatic response when it occurred. I soon learned that this is a national characteristic. The default self-presentation of New Zealanders is one of cheerful unflappability. "She'll be right," they say. No worries. It will all work out.

In one of my early conversations with Ron Jones, I asked him what had moved him to join the fight to expose the unfortunate experiment. His answer was matter-of-fact: "The reason I got involved was that it was wrong that women were unnecessarily getting cancer and dying. That was wrong."

Then Jones pointed to the values that he shared with McIndoe. "And so my Presbyterian background said, 'Ron, you'd better get involved.' It's probably a reflection of the nature of the man I am. I wasn't prepared to sit down and pretend I didn't know about it. Which is what all my colleagues did."

Jones didn't explain exactly what Presbyterian values he was referring to, but he didn't really need to. I come from a long line of Presbyterians on my mother's side. I grew up in the Presbyterian Church, went to Presbyterian Sunday School, and graduated from a college founded by Presbyterians. My best friends as a child were Presbyterians. So were my worst enemies. My maternal grandmother and grandfather were not just regular-army Presbyterians but Associate Reformed Presbyterians, which is like the special forces branch of the Presbyterian Church: stricter, more hard-nosed, and even less fun. Other denominations refer to Presbyterians as "the frozen Chosen." I have slept through so many Presbyterian sermons that to this day I nod off at the mere mention of the Book of Romans.

The Dunedin variant of Presbyterianism is largely a secular one, stripped of its harsh theological underpinnings and softened by a South Pacific climate. New Zealand is a tolerant country, its culture deeply influenced by the communitarian values of the Māori. Most New Zealanders are far too good-humored to nurse a grudge with the care and devotion of the South Carolina Presbyterians I grew up with. Yet the Presbyterians who came to Dunedin from Scotland left a cultural mark that struck me as very familiar.

It is probably fair to say that Presbyterians are not widely known for their sense of playful joy. We are known for our grim stoicism, our constipated emotional lives, and our complicated attitudes toward money. When the word "Presbyterian" is used as a noun, the adjective that most often precedes it is "staid." Presbyterians pride themselves on their traditions of frugality, dutiful service, and self-restraint. Not long ago, Ina and I met up with a group of my former classmates from David-son College, a liberal arts college established by Presbyterians in North Carolina. We were waiting in line to get into a bas-ketball tournament when a limo pulled up. A group of drunk Auburn fans spilled out yelling "Go War Eagles!" We all stared silently at our shoes. Ina looked around and asked, "Come on, where are all the 'Go Davidson!' cheers?" An older man wear-ing a Davidson sweater turned around and said quietly, "There will be cheering." He paused. "It will be respectful."

This may not sound like the ideal training ground for future whistleblowers. And it must be admitted that the aver-age Presbyterian is less likely to march in a protest or topple a statue than to write a strongly worded letter to the editor. Nor in my experience are Presbyterians any less inclined than oth-ers to hypocrisy, sanctimony, grudge holding, or all-around sinful behavior. But Presbyterians do have one characteristic that lends itself well to whistleblowing, and that is our stub-bornness, especially when it comes to matters of principle. We don't compromise easily and we don't give up, not even when reason, mercy, and common sense say that we should.

Non-Presbyterians have informed me that obstinacy is not universally seen as a virtue. It can lead to self-righteous mor-alizing, festering grievances, and the relentless pursuit of ill-advised causes. The steadfast Confederate General Stonewall Jackson was a Presbyterian who owned slaves. John Knox, the Scottish Jeremiah and founder of the Presbyterian Church in Scotland, was a well-known misogynist whose most famous publication was called "The First Blast of the Trumpet against the Monstrous Regiment of Women."[31] Yet Knox, like Jackson, was nothing if not tenacious. He fought against Catholicism and declared that a single celebration of the mass was worse than a cup of poison.[32] Mary Queen of Scots called him the most dangerous man in the kingdom.[33] Knox survived treason charges and assassination attempts and once served nineteen months chained to an oar as a French galley slave.[34] His grave, which now lies under an Edinburgh parking lot, is said to have been marked with the words, "Here lies one who neither flattered nor feared any flesh."[35]

Tenacity is a valuable trait for a whistleblower, where success often depends on perseverance against long odds. Bill McIndoe fought against the unfortunate experiment for twenty years. It took Martha Stephens even longer to get any measure of justice for the victims of the Cincinnati radiation experiments. Peter Buxtun spent nearly seven years trying to stop the forty-year Tuskegee syphilis study, and he wasn't even the first to try. Complicating the whistleblower's battle is the unfortunate fact that it is often unclear whether victory has been achieved. It wouldn't be unfair to say that Ron Jones, now in his eighties, is still fighting his own personal battle against the unfortunate experiment, more than three decades after the Cartwright Report was issued.

Of course, the great handicap that saddles Presbyterian whistleblowers is their sense of propriety. Just as we don't speak in tongues or clap in church, we don't enjoy making a public spectacle of ourselves. It feels so unseemly. And yet, making a public spectacle is often exactly what whistleblowing requires. In fact, it is essential to the mission. As Jones eventually learned, it is only when the ugliness of a scandal is publicly exposed that the public can be motivated to fix it.

• • •

When Ron Jones joined the staff of National Women's as a tutor specialist in the summer of 1973, he was self-conscious of his status as a newcomer. After spending the previous six years training in England, he had become the first physician from outside the hospital to be appointed to his position. "I was a total outsider," he says. An avid cricketer, Jones remembers being invited to play in a friendly match between the staff of National Women's and that of the neighboring Greenlane Hospital. Herb Green played too, wearing (it was rumored) the same cricket boots he had worn as a student at Otago. Wives and girlfriends served cucumber sandwiches and tea.

Jones was eager to develop his skills in colposcopy, so he approached Bill McIndoe, the hospital's expert. The two men took to each other immediately, even though McIndoe was old enough to be Jones's father. "I liked him because he had fun. He was a fun-loving man," Jones says, surprising me a little. "When visiting dignitaries came to New Zealand, parties were always held at our place. McIndoe would come and drink orange juice; his wife would run out the back and get a glass of gin with my wife; and I'd have a beer." Jones says McIndoe used to call him "Ronnie, my boy." "And I hated 'Ronnie,'" Jones says. "He was the only person who got away with calling me 'Ronnie, my boy.'"

For a time, Jones simply observed the conflict between Green and McIndoe. He was more sympathetic to McIndoe by virtue of their friendship, but Green had spent his career working on CIS. He was a senior figure who could be quite warmhearted with his patients. Once, when a young woman with advanced cervical cancer was too ill to attend her graduation, Green arranged for a private ceremony in the ward, where the woman was "capped" by the university vice-chancellor. The occasion was celebrated with tea and cakes.[36] Some colleagues appreciated Green's eccentricities. In his early days of practice, Green embarked on a crusade to sterilize the stray cats on hospital grounds. Nurses would prepare a surgical tray; medical students would round up stray cats; and Green would spay them in the operating room, instructing students to kill escaping fleas with ethyl chloride.[37]

Jones says there was no single event that persuaded him to take sides, but he remembers attending a conference cel-

ebrating the silver jubilee of the postgraduate school, where
McIndoe and Green both presented papers about the same
series of patients. "Green presented his series, which had a
1 percent cancer rate, and McIndoe presented his, which had
I think a 17 percent cancer rate," Jones says. "And nobody
questioned this difference. There were gynecologists from the
whole country." Jones shakes his head in amazement. "This is
the problem," he says. "Do you not have the courage to stand
up and say, 'There's an inconsistency here. Why is it? Please
explain'"? Nobody in the room asked that question. "They
just went to lunch," Jones says.

In 1976, when Green was away on an overseas trip, Jones
was asked to take care of a patient he calls "Phoebe," who had
been seen at National Women's since 1962.[38] Right away it
was clear that Green had badly mismanaged her care. "That
was my first contact with one of Green's patients, and she was
dying in front of me," Jones says. Over a period of years Green
had watched a premalignant condition extend to cover Phoebe's entire vulva, vagina, and perianal region. In 1974, when
McLean's pathology report indicated malignancy, Green had
simply written his disagreement on the report by hand. Two
years later, when Jones saw Phoebe, the bleeding from her
tumor was so extensive that she had to be transfused with
twelve units of blood. Jones was forced to operate, but the
surgery was only palliative. Phoebe had trusted Green completely even as he was botching her care. "I thought of my
mother," Jones says. "Because if my mother had lived in Auckland and she had that problem, she would have trusted Green
in the same way as Phoebe had."

In 1978, McIndoe presented his findings about CIS at a
major international conference in Florida. In attendance was
Dick Mattingly, the editor of *Obstetrics and Gynecology*, the
most prestigious specialist journal in the field. When Mattingly invited McIndoe to submit his study, McIndoe agreed

and asked McLean to be a coauthor. Yet the two men struggled to put a paper together. Mattingly pressed hard, telling McIndoe that he considered it a "landmark report." McIndoe kept making excuses, but he couldn't tell Mattingly the real problem, which, according to Jones, was "his lack of confidence and constant need for reassurance."[39] After four years of prodding, Mattingly finally asked McIndoe to bring in another author. McIndoe decided on Jones.

As a much younger man, Jones proved to be the catalyst that the collaboration needed. "My personality is quite different," Jones says. "I'm more of an 'action man.' I'm just the opposite of Bill there. He was a lovely, kind, soft, gentle fatherly figure. Whereas I said, 'Oh, you know, we've got to get this thing finished.'" Jones insisted on two conditions: first, he wanted to verify all the patient records for himself; and second, he wanted to bring an expert statistician on board, Peter Mullins, of Auckland University.

The study they eventually sent to Mattingly was convincing but complicated.[40] It compared two groups of patients with CIS over time. Group 1 consisted of women whose follow-up cervical smears after their management by hospital doctors showed no sign of disease. Group 2 consisted of women who continued to have abnormal cervical smears, irrespective of how they had been managed. Most of these women were the subjects in Green's experiment. The comparison showed that only 1.5 percent of the women in Group 1 developed invasive cancer in a period ranging from five to twenty-eight years, as compared to 22 percent of the women in Group 2. This meant that the women with continuing abnormal cervical smears had twenty-five times greater risk of developing cancer. According to Jones, the study told two stories: first, the familiar one that CIS often naturally developed into invasive cancer, and two, the story of "the disastrous outcomes for some women from whom treatment was deliberately withheld."[41]

The journal finally accepted the paper. "We were worried right to the last minute that somehow Bonham would stop publication," Jones says. "We really believed that in our heart—that he had the ability to stop publication." Indeed, Bonham appears to have given that possibility some thought. In 1982, after hearing a rumor that McIndoe was working on the paper, Bonham wrote to the medical superintendent asking him to investigate the paper, since "any publication emanating from this hospital must be acceptable to the hospital before it is submitted for publication, as I'm sure you'll agree."[42] Nothing came of Bonham's effort, but the three men did not relax until they got a cable from Mattingly saying, "It's been printed. It's being sent out to the world tomorrow."

Obstetrics and Gynecology published the paper in October 1984 with the inauspicious title, "The Invasive Potential of Carcinoma in Situ of the Cervix."[43] It was the lead article. The authors distributed copies to all the members of the senior medical staff. "And I was given the job of giving it to Bonham," Jones says. "I stood somewhat in fear of him, because he was such a fearsome man. I said something like, 'Well, you are aware that Dr. McIndoe and I were writing a paper about carcinoma in situ, and the results of the management of carcinoma in situ. I think you should read it and act appropriately.'" Bonham was polite, but he did not comment.

With the publication of their paper, McIndoe, McLean, and Jones had lit the fuse on an explosive. All that remained was to grip the arms of their chairs and wait. Yet the paper was met with utter silence. It got no response from the authorities at National Women's Hospital, no response from hospital colleagues, and no response from the wider medical community. After years of slow, agonizing work, McIndoe, McLean, and Jones had not changed anyone's opinions in the slightest. The three men were bewildered. According to Jones, "It seemed incomprehensible to us that no one said anything."

The men had made a common mistake. Many reluctant whistleblowers feel deep obligations of loyalty to their institution. Yes, they want the wrongdoing to stop, but they don't want to bring the institution crashing down. The last thing they want is to air their dirty laundry in public. Like good Presbyterians, they are reluctant to make a spectacle of themselves. And so they work for years in quiet desperation, repeating the same failed strategies, trying every possible tactic except for the unthinkable one that might actually work, which is taking their story to the press.

• • •

Sandra Coney first heard rumors of the upcoming paper a year before it was published. Coney was the editor of *Broadsheet*, a feminist magazine, and she had a friend who worked with Peter Mullins, the statistician. Mullins had described the paper as "dynamite." But when it finally arrived in her mailbox in October 1984, Coney found it hard to decipher. It didn't look like dynamite. The numbers were disturbing, but there was no hint that the authors found the study unethical. In fact, Coney mistakenly assumed that McIndoe, McLean, and Jones had experimented on the women themselves and were now publishing their results.[44]

Coney sent a copy of the paper to Phillida Bunkle, a fellow feminist activist and a lecturer in women's studies at Victoria University, in Wellington. Along with other members of a women's health advocacy group, Fertility Action, they wrote to the authors with questions. The reply they got was unhelpful. McIndoe, still wary of the press, said they had misunderstood the study and he couldn't answer their questions. "We were very suspicious of the feminists," Jones says. "They were very suspicious of us." None of the men were quite ready to embrace the role of whistleblower. Far better for someone from the outside to point a finger at Green.

Two years later, that person came forward. Clare Matheson, a deputy principal at an Auckland girls' school, was a former patient of Green's who had developed invasive cervical cancer in 1985. She had undergone a hysterectomy as well as agonizing radiation treatments. Matheson had no idea she had ever been part of a study until Coney, who had heard about Matheson through a mutual friend, sent her a copy of the paper. Matheson was stunned. As she read it, she felt a rushing sound in her ears. Matheson told her friend, "I was a guinea pig."[45]

When Matheson first visited National Women's Hospital in 1964, she was a twenty-seven-year-old mother of three. Her general practitioner had examined her several weeks after a miscarriage and found a suspicious cervical smear. He referred her to National Women's, where Green examined her. Her diagnosis was carcinoma in situ, but Green did not remove the lesion.[46] And when Green was given the green light to begin the unfortunate experiment two years later, Matheson was one of the subjects he enrolled.

Over the next fifteen years, Matheson visited National Women's Hospital thirty-four times. She had twenty-eight cervical smears, ten colposcopic examinations, five biopsies, and four surgical procedures under general anesthetic.[47] Although Matheson was told repeatedly that she should not worry about cancer, Matheson couldn't help but wonder why she was being subjected to so many examinations and biopsies. Once, when she saw Green, she suggested that perhaps she was being used as a guinea pig. Green did not appreciate the remark. "'You'll do as you're told,' he said loudly, his face flushed with anger," Matheson remembered. "It is difficult to respond to that kind of comment when one is flat on one's back and half-clothed. I lay there feeling like a chastised child."[48] When Green discharged her from his care in 1979, he wrote in her file, "I do not think any further active follow-up is needed."[49] Yet nine of her pathology or histology reports over the fifteen-year period were marked "conclusive for malignancy."[50]

Matheson was angry enough to speak to Coney and Bunkle on the record. The two reporters also found a key informant in Jock McLean, who had done away with whatever reservations he once had about talking to the press. Virtually the first thing McLean said to Coney and Bunkle when they came to his office was, "What took you fellows so long?" They warmed to McLean right away, despite his habit of referring to women as "females." He was an unusual man, Coney writes, even a little lordly, but forthright and caring. McLean asked if it was true they were feminists. "Yes," they told him, wondering how he would react. "How bad are you?" McLean asked. "As bad as they come," Coney replied.[51]

McLean knew Clare Matheson's case file by heart. "People in the tea room talked about Matheson and said how terrible it is," McLean told Coney. "They'll say it behind Herb's back, but they won't confront him."[52] McLean had been fighting with Green for years. Although Green had no formal qualifications as a pathologist, he had an infuriating habit of substituting his own diagnosis for McLean's on the glass pathology slides. "Herb's an absolute bastard when stood up to," McLean said. "Most people were frightened of him. When McIndoe and I tried to stand up to him, he reacted by doing nothing and saying nothing. He's a bigoted zealot. He's like a missionary who thinks he can do no wrong."[53]

Coney and Bunkle published their report in the June 1987 issue of *Metro* magazine under the title "An Unfortunate Experiment at National Women's." In the very first sentence, a patient named "Ruth"—later identified as Clare Matheson— compared an appointment at National Women's to a visit to Auschwitz. Yet most media outlets ignored the *Metro* story, and for several days it appeared as if it might suffer the same fate as the 1984 paper. That changed dramatically on June 4, when Peter Kingston, of Radio New Zealand, broadcast an interview with Clare Matheson and the president of the Auckland Cancer Society came out in favor of a public inquiry.[54] With that, the dam broke. Every media outlet in the country leaped to cover the story. On June 10, the Minister of Health announced a public inquiry to be led by Judge Silvia Cartwright, a respected district court judge with a record of work on women's issues.[55]

In ordinary circumstances, this might have been a victory. But it didn't feel that way to Ron Jones. Ten months earlier, in September 1986, Bill McIndoe had died unexpectedly of a heart condition. When the *Metro* article was published in June, many of Jones's colleagues saw it as a betrayal and abandoned him. Worst of all, Jones was dealing with the devastating news that his wife, Barbara, had metastatic breast cancer. They were the parents of four children. Jones would go on to testify in the Cartwright Inquiry, but with his wife undergoing chemotherapy and an uncertain future looming, he didn't have much strength for the task. It would be left to Green's victims and colleagues to reveal the full extent of the wrongdoing at National Women's.

• • •

It's March 18, 2020, and the sun is out at a farmhouse in the bush south of Auckland. I'm sitting outside with Ron Jones and Michael Churchouse, the former head of the cytology laboratory at National Women's. Churchouse is eighty-seven years old now, thin as a reed and a little frail. He's wearing a Lancer cap, a flannel shirt, and baggy trousers held up by suspenders. "That dog's an absolute disgrace," Churchouse says, pointing to a scraggly white mutt lurking nearby. "Last night she put up a possum somewhere." Above us is a trellis lined with vines so thick I could reach up and pick the grapes, but what I keep reaching for instead is the large bottle of hand sanitizer sitting nearby. It is there courtesy of Churchouse's son, Dave, who has been spooked by the recent arrival of the coronavirus to New Zealand. Churchouse rolls his eyes as Dave hovers in the background making certain we all sit at least 6 feet apart. "Sorry," Churchouse says. "He takes it very seriously."

Jones and I are here to talk to Churchouse about the Cartwright Inquiry. Public hearings began on August 3, 1987, less than two months after the *Metro* article was published, and they continued for six months. The press gave them wall-to-wall coverage. Twelve patients and two relatives gave evidence publicly; a further seventy gave evidence privately. Medical advisers for the inquiry reviewed over twelve hundred patient files.[56] Green, Bonham, and other hospital physicians and administrators were forced to defend their actions. Each day seemed to bring another jaw-dropping abuse. Churchouse appeared before the inquiry in November. "I was a bit of a whistleblower," he says.

Churchouse's revelations came in response to questioning. He was asked about some cytology smears ordered by Herb Green. Strangely, these smears came from newborn girls. "From where physically were these smears taken?" asked the attorney. "The vaginal vault," Churchouse replied, to astonished stares. As part of a research study begun by Green in 1963, nurses had performed "vaginal swabs" on more than twenty-two hundred baby girls.[57] This procedure involved opening a baby's vagina and inserting a moist cotton swab to sample vaginal cells without the knowledge or consent of the parents. The rationale lay in Green's theory of CIS. Green suspected that many infant girls were born with abnormal cells in their vaginas that would never turn cancerous. If true, this finding might lend credence to his belief that CIS was benign. Green was wrong, of course, and when that became apparent, he lost interest in the study. But nobody told the nurses, who continued to collect the swabs as a matter of routine for over two and a half years.[58]

No babies were harmed, but the public was outraged. An *Auckland Star* editorial called the study "sick, the vilest practice yet revealed at an inquiry which had uncovered some gross practices."[59] At first Green claimed that nurses had collected only two hundred swabs and that their purpose was to detect gonorrhea. But these claims were easily proven false. "I had kept all these requests, the slides, everything," Churchouse says. He had put them in apple boxes and stored them in a crawl space. When his claim about the vaginal swabs was challenged, Churchouse knew just what to do. "I said, I'll show you them! And I'll show you the forms!" says Churchouse, his voice rising. "They just about had a fit, didn't they? Of course, it was what, thirty, forty years old? And I'd saved this bloody thing. Because I'm a pack rat by nature."

The so-called "baby smear" scandal was not the only unexpected revelation. There was also the "flying uterus" case. Green had taken several excised uteruses with him on a plane to New York without having them biopsied first. One uterus was positive for malignancy, and the patient's cancer diagnosis was delayed for months.[60] The inquiry also found that physicians and trainees had performed vaginal exams and practiced inserting IUDs on anesthetized, unconscious women without their consent or knowledge. Dennis Bonham defended the practice, explaining that asking permission from the women would be too time-consuming and expensive.[61] That explanation did not play well with the public. The Human Rights Commissioner called the practice a "form of rape," and the Minister of Health ordered hospital boards to make sure the practice was stopped.[62]

As we talk, Dave keeps popping by to make sure we are abiding by the COVID safety procedures. I'm grateful for his vigilance. The very last thing I want to do is unintentionally infect two men in their eighties with COVID. But Churchouse and Jones seem unfazed. When Churchouse retired from National

Women's at the age of sixty, he and his wife set sail on a 30-foot wooden boat and spent the next seven years at sea. During that time, they were placed under house arrest in Russia and escaped hostile gunfire off the coast of Yemen.[63] Churchouse tells me his proudest voyage was to an uninhabited archipelago nearly 300 miles south of New Zealand's South Island. "I did it with just a plastic sextant and a radio—a cheap one—and a compass," he says. Jones adds, "That's why New Zealanders were the first to climb Everest. They're a bit of a mad lot."

When Churchouse recalls his epic battles with Herb Green, a glint of mischief appears in his eyes. "Green and I used to have shouting matches at times," Churchouse says. "He was a bully. He was a natural bully, old Green." I feel like Jim Hawkins at the Admiral Benbow, listening to an aging pirate. When Churchouse was called into the hospital on urgent matters, he'd sometimes pull his car into a space reserved exclusively for doctors. Green would poke his head out and shout, "You can't park there!" Churchouse would shout back, "Well, I am!" On one occasion at a party, Green told Churchouse, "You know, Michael, I'll be remembered when I die. You won't be." I ask Churchouse what the context for the remark was. "Drinking," he replies.

"He was always undermining cytology as an arm of medical science, which, you know, we took seriously," Churchouse says. A long-standing battle concerned Green's habit of writing his own diagnostic opinions on top of those of the trained cytology staff. If Green disagreed with the results, he would simply write in his own diagnosis. Churchouse says he finally had rubber stamps made that were so large Green couldn't write over them. I ask if the stamps were specifically for the purpose of stopping Green. "Shit, yes!" he says. "This was war!" Churchouse says they used to keep all the files that were positive for malignancy in a file marked "D." As it happened, D was also the name of the academic clinical team that included Green. When new staff members joined the cytology lab, they would ask, "Why is that file marked D?" The answer was, "D for Dead," Churchouse says. "Because those were all Green's patients."

The Cartwright Report left no doubt that McIndoe, McLean, and Jones had been vindicated. Green had not performed well under scrutiny. By the time he testified at the inquiry, he was seventy-one years old and in poor health, yet he still managed to patronize the attorneys questioning him, suggesting at one point that they were incapable of understanding the medical terms he employed. He denied making a comment attributed to him in the *Metro* article but was forced to back down when a recording was produced.[64] Cartwright found not only that Green had failed to obtain proper informed consent and given his patients inadequate treatment for CIS, but that evidence also suggested he had manipulated his research data. If not for his failing health, he would have almost certainly been sanctioned by the New Zealand Medical Council.

Dennis Bonham had fared little better. Some observers found him evasive and disingenuous. Clare Matheson compared him to Toad in *Wind in the Willows*. "When he thought he had said anything smart, clever or witty, he would glance at the judge and give her an ingratiating grin, like a Third Former looking for more marks," she writes.[65] Cartwright subjected Bonham to withering criticism in the report, noting his misleading comments, his lack of impartiality as chair of the Ethical Committee at National Women's, and his failure to stop Green's study. The Medical Council eventually found Bonham guilty of seven misconduct charges, including five charges of disgraceful conduct.[66]

Two years after McIndoe died, the Cartwright Report finally provided authoritative confirmation that he had been right all along. "I have been left with the eerie impression that

Dr McIndoe's various memoranda and notes were almost pro-
phetic," Cartwright wrote.[67] Yet McIndoe was a prophet without honor in his own community. In 1966, McIndoe had been
the sole voice of dissent against Green's study. It took years
before he was joined by McLean and Jones, and even with the
support of other staff members, such as Michael Churchouse,
their small group never constituted more than a tiny minority
within the hospital. Everyone else sided with Green. How
could that possibly happen?

• • •

The word "groupthink" has become such a cliché for bad collective decision-making that it's easy to forget its intellectual
history. The sociologist William Whyte coined the term in
Fortune magazine in 1952. Whyte explained that by "groupthink" he was not referring to instinctive conformity, which is
a familiar failing, but "rationalized conformity," which doesn't
see conformity as a failing at all. Rationalized conformity is an
"open, articulate philosophy which holds that group values
are not only expedient but right and good as well."[68] It isn't
just that individuals are looking too eagerly at others rather
than consulting their own moral compasses. It's that getting
along with others has replaced every external purpose. For
Whyte, the true appeal of belonging to groups is simple: they
give us freedom from moral choice.

Whyte went on to write *The Organization Man* in 1956,
which stands alongside Sloan Wilson's novel *The Man in the
Gray Flannel Suit* and David Riesman's *The Lonely Crowd* as
that decade's best-known indictments of postwar social conformity. But it was the Yale social psychologist Irving Janis
who did the most to turn "groupthink" into an object of formal academic study. What triggered the idea for his 1972
book, *Victims of Groupthink*, was reading Arthur Schlesinger's
account of the Bay of Pigs fiasco in *A Thousand Days*. "How

could bright, shrewd men like John F. Kennedy and his advisors be taken in by the CIA's stupid, patchwork plan?" Janis wondered.[69] When he put the Bay of Pigs invasion alongside other disastrous policy decisions, Janis saw a pattern. Not only did the terrible decisions come from cohesive groups, but the cohesion also appeared to make their decisions worse.

That cohesion is worse than antagonism might seem implausible. All of us, especially those of us who work in universities, understand the grinding frustration of working in dysfunctional groups. According to Janis, however, the opposite is no better. Cohesive groups, he argued, produce "mindless conformity and collective misjudgment of serious risks, which are collectively laughed off in a collective atmosphere of clubby conviviality."[70] The conformity comes not from authoritarian enforcement but from the soft power of belonging. In cohesive groups, everyone feels less anxious and more secure. They enjoy the company of one another and share a sense of common purpose. It is exactly this easy amiability that discourages independent thought and dissenting views, especially if those views threaten the cohesiveness of the group.

Whether Janis is right about cohesive groups is debatable. One of the case studies he offers up is the Watergate cover-up. Yet the Nixon White House was hardly a model of "clubby conviviality." It was an incubator for paranoia, suspicion, and self-serving flattery of the president. But Janis is certainly right to highlight the pleasures of social conformity. Collaborators in wrongdoing often defend their failure to break ranks by saying they were terrified of the consequences. But they rarely admit what all of us know in our hearts, which is that the terrifying consequence is often nothing more than being disliked. Not many of us will take a hard moral stand if it means sacrificing the respect and appreciation of our friends.

As the Cartwright Report suggests, the work culture at

National Women's was complex. It was neither a place of clubby conviviality nor one of hostile dysfunction. It is true that many staff members found Green difficult. Yet Green was good friends with the leading lights at National Women's, Bill Liley and Graham "Mont" Liggins. Not only did Green collaborate on scientific papers with Liley and Liggins, but they also owned a forestry venture together. The scientific work of Liley and Liggins had given National Women's its sterling reputation. Liley performed the world's first intrauterine blood transfusion, while Liggins pioneered the use of corticosteroid injections to accelerate the lung growth of premature infants. Both men would eventually be knighted for their contributions to medicine. Neither of them had any reason to fear Green, yet neither of them opposed the "unfortunate experiment."[71] Many years later, Liggins would admit that he and Liley had turned a blind eye to it.[72]

One possible reason for the absence of open dissent at National Women's is self-deception. According to *Exit, Voice, and Loyalty,* Albert Hirschman's famous book on organizational dissent, the more difficult it is to get into an organization, the higher the degree of self-deception there will be within the organization. When members pay a high entrance fee, literally or metaphorically, they have a higher stake in proving they made a good decision to join.[73] The members of elite organizations are loyal. They defend the organization to others. They find the organization's activities interesting and valuable, no matter how boring they are. And when things in elite organizations go bad, as they did at National Women's, the members of the organization will be the last to recognize it.

A second reason may have been the rigid status system. "I couldn't believe the hierarchy," says Mary Whaley, who worked in the sterile supply department at National Women's as a university student. To join the staff of National Women's was to find yourself in a medieval cosmology as hierarchical as the Great Chain of Being. At the very top, striding the hallway like gods, were the physicians. Below them, in descending order, were nurses and technicians, and below them the cooks and cleaners. Although McIndoe, McLean, and Jones ranked well above the lowly nurses, they were still "visiting" staff members and thus lower in status than the academic staff. According to Jones, this was the main reason they were not taken seriously. As an attorney at the Cartwright Inquiry later put it, McIndoe's objections to Green's study were "equivalent to the office boy trying to tell the managing director how to run the firm."[74]

According to Irving Janis, the force of social conformity is especially powerful in institutions that are driven by a deep sense of moral purpose. In academic health centers, that moral purpose is embedded in the dogma that medical research saves lives. When McIndoe questioned Green's research, he was challenging everything that academic medicine sees as righteous and holy. Such challenges demand a harsh response, even if the moral cost is high. As Janis writes, "'Since our group's objectives are good,' the members feel, 'any means we decide to use must be good.' This shared assumption helps members avoid the feelings of shame or guilt about decisions that may violate their code of ethical behavior."[75]

When dissenters emerge, according to Janis, they are handled in predictable ways. One strategy is to "domesticate" the dissenter. The term was coined by James C. Thomson, a member of the Lyndon Johnson administration during the Vietnam War. Thomson explained that the Johnson cabinet neutralized doubters not by bullying or excluding them, but by making them feel at home in the group despite their dissent. This strategy brought cohesion to the group and satisfied the moral demands of dissenters, who could rest easier knowing that they had spoken out.[76]

More often members of the group will try valiantly to convince dissenters to change their minds. If that doesn't work, they may cajole the dissenter into compromising or meeting them halfway. If even that fails, the group will simply stop communicating with the dissenter entirely. "The members begin to exclude him, often quite subtly at first and later more obviously, in order to restore the unity of the group," Janis writes.[77] Once the group has silenced or exiled the dissenter, everyone can relax, comfortable once again that their beliefs won't be challenged. All three dissenters at National Women's felt this kind of exclusion, even Jock McLean. "I kept away from the clinicians. I felt an antipathy against me," he told Coney and Bunkle. "They feared I was opening my mouth too wide."[78]

• • •

In March of 2020, as I was finishing up a visit to Auckland, Ron Jones told me about an unsettling encounter over the Christmas holidays. Jones and his partner, Loris, were waiting for a performance of Handel's Messiah. Across the room Jones noticed a stranger who kept glancing over at him. It made Jones self-conscious. Eventually, the stranger sidled up to him and said, "So you're the bastard who caused all that trouble at National Women's." Jones told the story with resignation rather than bitterness. This is simply what his life is like now.

In a just world, Jones could feel proud of what he did. The Cartwright Inquiry was arguably the most comprehensive and successful investigation of a medical research scandal in the modern era. The reforms that were instituted in its wake have been remarkably effective. In the thirty-odd years since the Cartwright Report was released—a period that has seen shameful abuses of human subjects in other countries—New Zealand has not experienced a single major research scandal. In comparison with virtually every other research whistleblower, Jones won a stunning victory. Why does that victory feel so much like a failure?

"Even today as we sit here talking, I feel guilty—and I know I shouldn't—that I caused all that trouble," Jones says, remembering the Cartwright Inquiry. "I mean, people say to me, 'You should have a knighthood for this, Ron,' or, 'You should wear this as a badge of honor.' Whereas in fact, it's been a terrible emotional burden on me which I feel to this day. I feel I've made quite a lot of worthwhile contributions in the field of women's health and education, science, and so on. But they're all forgotten. I'm just remembered as someone who caused all that trouble."

As a rule, New Zealanders are not given to introspection. They are pragmatic, outward-looking people, more comfortable speaking about winds and weather patterns than their inner psychological turmoil. When Jones speaks about his past actions, he has the sound of an honorable man peering at himself in puzzlement from the outside. He doesn't consider his whistleblowing heroic or even morally exceptional. He simply felt ashamed of what he saw happening to patients and tried to make it right. He believes the others at National Women's should have done the same as a matter of duty. While Jones says he feels guilty about his actions, he also feels the need to defend them vigorously against those who criticize him. His sensitivity is understandable. He lives in a small country with an even smaller medical community. Judgment is not easy to escape.

In the world of honor, whether you feel pride or shame depends crucially on the judgment of your community. To feel proud of an action requires the good opinions of the people you respect. If those people condemn your actions, your instinctive response is shame. And the very possibility of righteous rebellion against that community—to assert that you are right, regardless of what others say—depends on loyalty to moral ideals that stand apart from the community values you believe are wrong. It means being true to your conscience, the authentic self that lies behind your social role.

Jones speaks about his choice as a matter of conscience and character. What he did was simply a reflection of who he was. Jones, McIndoe, and McLean had all grown up in working-class families. "We had very simple, working-class values, which I think had great value in this situation," Jones tells me. "You don't get complicated with the bullshit." When Jones first went to National Women's, he was proud to be a part of an institution that had made such significant contributions to the care of women. "Very proud, and I still am. But nonetheless, I'm ashamed of what happened," Jones says. "I felt a tinge of sorrow for Bonham and Green who had gotten themselves in such a mess." He also feels ashamed of the medical community, especially the people who stayed silent. Occasionally, he'll get a call from a doctor who wants to talk. "They usually want to talk about themselves, though," he says. "They are rationalizing why they didn't get involved."

In *Exit, Voice, and Loyalty*, Albert Hirschman contrasts two different responses to what he calls "organizational decline."[79] By decline, Hirschman has in mind a range of situations where things in an organization are going bad, from poor performance to ethical abuses. Hirschman calls the two responses to decline "exit" and "voice." Exit is typically found in the realm of economics. You express dissent in the economic realm by buying your goods elsewhere or selling your stock in a company. Voice belongs to the realm of politics. You express dissent in the political realm by voting, speaking out, or protesting. With either response, exit or voice, your hope is that the expression of dissent will arrest the decline of the organization and fix the problem at hand.

To most Americans, exit is the obvious choice. Why would anyone stay at an organization in decline, especially if that organization is a hospital where patients are being mistreated? According to Hirschman, an important development that amplified exit as a possible response was the consumer rights movement of the 1960s. If you are unhappy with a product or a service, you simply shop elsewhere. The same goes for decline in public schools, universities, churches, or political parties. In America, the natural solution to a problem is the exit door.

Loyalty puts a check on exit as an option. The more loyal to an organization the members are, the more likely they are to try to fix the organization rather than simply leave it. There's a reason why many Catholics horrified at the sexual abuse scandals in the Catholic Church don't simply leave and become Episcopalians or Methodists. They feel a duty to fix the problem. In fact, they may feel that duty even more acutely than someone on the outside, simply because it's their church. Exit feels a lot like surrender. It's hard to see how an exit from National Women's would have helped any of the mistreated research subjects, which may be why none of the dissenters left. McIndoe, McLean, and Jones all stayed at the hospital until retirement or death.

Jones says the atmosphere at National Women's turned poisonous as soon as the Cartwright Inquiry was announced. "Everything changed. I remember walking into the hospital on a Monday morning. Groups of people were standing in the corridors and when they saw me coming, there was a hushed silence," Jones says. "And then of course I had colleagues who said they would never speak to me again or work with me again, that sort of thing." Jones was taken aback by the response. "Well, I must say naively I thought my colleagues would support me, knowing that they didn't really believe Herb anyhow," he says. Even the colleagues who didn't confront him directly made him feel awkward. "I felt that once you're a whistleblower, your colleagues may not be friends, but they certainly don't want to be seen associating with you.

For example, I stopped going to the Hospital Medical Committee meetings because it was so bloody unpleasant. They were still whinging why the Cartwright Report had come out so badly against the hospital. If I was sitting there, it was just too uncomfortable. So I began to avoid situations that I knew would cause tension for me."

What made that period even more traumatic for Jones was the illness of his wife, who would eventually die of breast cancer. "This was terrible because Barbara was having chemotherapy. I had a young family, and life was shit, and I knew I had to keep working. I was in my mid-forties at this stage, so I was still pretty young," Jones says. "Of course, we tried to shield the kids." Jones pauses for a long time. It is hard for him to talk about this episode without getting tearful. Our conversation has ripped open an old wound. "It was just terrible. Unbelievably terrible," he says. "And I had to face the inquiry. And I really just didn't have the strength to do it."

Jones and I are speaking about the ordeal over coffee and homemade tea loaf in his sitting room. Jones lives in a spacious house overlooking Hobson's Bay, all giant windows and open spaces. Surrounding the house are lush, subtropical plants—king fern, cabbage trees, banana, tamarillo. Jones has planted a vegetable garden next to the garage. Several of his children live nearby, and his partner, Loris, a retired schoolteacher, is a ferry ride away on the island of Waiheki, in the Hauraki Gulf. Jones walks regularly along the bay, although his gait is slightly impaired from a trekking accident in the southern Alps that paralyzed him for a period and damaged his sense of proprioception. "I look like a boozer but I'm not," he says cheerfully.

I'm often struck by how upbeat Jones seems, despite his psychological wounds. His face is almost never without a smile. I feel sure his energy and optimism helped carry him through dark times at National Women's, yet I sometimes wonder if it is a strain. One reason I love New Zealand is the unrelenting optimism of New Zealanders. Their good cheer is infectious. Life always looks better in Dunedin. Yet I have never experienced anything deeply traumatic there. What would it be like to feel terrible in a culture that demands that you put the best face on misfortune, to feel bereft in a country that refuses to admit that the glass is ever half empty? It might make you feel even more alone in your sadness.

As comprehensive as the inquiry was, it did not settle the issue for good. In March 1989, less than a year after the Cartwright Report was published, a Wellington newspaper published an article with the headline "Cartwright Report Based on a Scam."[80] That was soon followed by a *Metro* article, "Second Thoughts on the Unfortunate Experiment," in which a staff writer characterized Green as the "victim of a well-orchestrated smear campaign" and Coney as a "feminist lobbyist" with a "well-documented loathing of male doctors."[81] Even today, the findings of the Cartwright Report are disputed. In 2012, describing Green's experiment as a "careful and open study" and the Cartwright Inquiry as a "mixture of farce and tragedy," Cambridge University researcher Robin Carrell asked, "How does an enlightened nation descend into irrationality and allow witch-hunts to destroy the lives of decent people?"[82] Sir Iain Chalmers, one of the founders of the Cochrane Collaboration, has even called for a prize honoring Herb Green.[83]

The most outspoken revisionist has been Auckland University historian Linda Bryder, whose book, *A History of the "Unfortunate Experiment" at National Women's Hospital*, was published in 2009.[84] Bryder contested virtually every major finding of the Cartwright Report. In her account, what Green did with CIS was not really research; it was conservative treatment. Not only that, but it was also treatment completely within the boundaries of accepted clinical practice at the time.

His failure to get informed consent from the women in the study was consistent with the ethical norms and codes of the period, such as the Declaration of Helsinki.[85] So was the practice of performing pelvic exams and procedures on unconscious women without their permission. "I came to realise there was no experimentation," Bryder told the *New Zealand Listener* magazine. "The decisions on treatment were based on clinical decisions by doctors doing the best they could for individual patients."[86]

For Jones, the main result of this revisionism is that the issue never goes away. "I'm the only living whistleblower. The others are all dead, and a new generation comes along and I'm kind of a public figure. If someone has a question to ask, a reporter, a granddaughter, whatever, it always comes to me," he says. Fortunately, Jones has not been entirely alone. Charlotte Paul, now retired from her position as head of the Department of Preventive Medicine at the University of Otago, has been a fierce defender of the Cartwright Report, as has Sir David Skegg, the originator of the phrase "unfortunate experiment," who went on to become vice-chancellor of the University of Otago. Historians such as Joanna Manning and Barbara Brookes have published scathing takedowns of Bryder's scholarship, most notably in the edited book *The Cartwright Papers.*[87]

In 2017, Jones published *Doctors in Denial,* his own book about the unfortunate experiment. It is a powerful account of the scandal and the first to come from a National Women's insider. Jones also called publicly for an apology to be offered to the victims of the experiment and their families. First he shamed the Royal Australian and New Zealand College of Obstetricians and Gynaecologists into apologizing.[88] A year later, he did the same for the Auckland District Health Board.[89] Jones even got an apology from Prime Minister Jacinda Ardern. He believes that Auckland University owes the women an apology as well, but the university disagrees. "All the way I've had to tell people to say, 'I'm sorry,' you know," Jones says. "Everybody who said, 'I'm sorry,' I had to go and say, 'You've got to say you're sorry.' Well, it wasn't my job to tell them. They should instinctively feel they're sorry."

At times I have gently suggested to Jones that he should simply declare victory and move on. For most New Zealanders, the matter is settled. I have reminded Jones how much more successful his struggle has been in comparison with that of other whistleblowers and activists, including me. But Jones doesn't see it that way. His view is more Presbyterian. Whenever there is a challenge to the record, no matter how marginal or ill conceived, he feels compelled to strike back. Sometimes I think he will never be satisfied until he has convinced every last New Zealander that he was right.

I once asked Jones, "Has anyone ever said, 'You were right, and I was wrong'?" He replied, "No, not a soul. Not a single soul. There were some people who were silently supportive. Those people did show their heads a bit after the inquiry. But none of them ever said to me what you've just said to me: 'Ron, you were right, and I should have done something about it.' It didn't happen like that. Nobody ever said, 'I was wrong.'" Jones doesn't think it is possible for him to move on. "I used to play a lot of cricket," Jones says. "And it was nice to have a good innings, to play a good innings and feel proud of yourself and say, 'That was a good innings, and we won the match.' Within a couple of days, that's history." But the unfortunate experiment never leaves him. "It can eat you from the inside," Jones says. "It will be with me to the grave."

CHAPTER 7

The Karolinska

Paolo Macchiarini relaxes into a barber's chair, leaning back to have his hair washed. "I am working for the university, and we are trying to create new organs," he tells the barber, pausing to add an explanation: "Frankenstein." Although Macchiarini is fending off charges of research misconduct at his university, he appears untroubled, even carefree, in this scene from Bosse Lindquist's documentary *The Experiments*.[1] Knowing what lies ahead for him—dismissal, disgrace, manslaughter charges—it's hard not to think of the beginning of Brian De Palma's film *The Untouchables*, in which Robert De Niro, playing Al Capone, entertains questions from reporters as he gets a shave. Macchiarini is just as charming. As the barber finishes his work, Macchiarini breaks into a mischievous grin. "Perfect," he says, clapping his hands in appreciation.

Few medical research scandals are as spectacular as those engineered by Paolo Macchiarini, a charismatic, Swiss-born transplant surgeon. Macchiarini made international headlines in 2008 when he performed the world's first trachea transplant in Spain. Two years later, he was invited to set up a research program at the Karolinska Institute, in Sweden. One of Europe's premier medical centers, the Karolinska Institute awards the Nobel Prize in Physiology or Medicine. There Macchiarini began implanting the world's first artificial tracheas into patients—and by his account, doing it with great success. But soon there were murmurs about his methods. His patients appeared to be dying. In 2015, an external expert commissioned by the Karolinska Institute found him guilty of research misconduct. Yet the leaders of the Karolinska continued to defend Macchiarini and dismissed allegations by his critics, including four of his colleagues. That defense crumbled in the early months of 2016, when Lindquist's riveting three-part documentary was shown on Swedish television. The ensuing scandal not only led to the dismissal of Macchiarini and the senior leadership of the institute, but also threatened the future of the Nobel Prize in Physiology or Medicine.

In the years since *The Experiments* aired, Macchiarini has been exposed as a medical con man unlike any other: a fabulist, a fraud, a globe-trotting Casanova who lied to women as smoothly as he did to his patients. Macchiarini concocted a false biography and published fraudulent scientific papers; he manipulated the press like a public relations professional. All this he did with such facility that he fooled experts at the highest levels of academic medicine. Like a cross between Christiaan Barnard and Bernie Madoff, Macchiarini used his charisma to exploit unwitting victims for years until *The Experiments* brought it all crashing down.

Rarely has a work of investigative reporting on a medical research scandal produced such devastating consequences. The only real rival is Sandra Coney and Phillida Bunkle's 1987 article in *Metro* magazine on the "unfortunate experiment" in Auckland. But the *Metro* article came well after Herb Green had retired. *The Experiments* caught Macchiarini in the act. What made the film so effective was not just the gruesome nature of the deaths it documented or even the eagerness of the Karolinska leaders to exonerate Macchiarini from blame, but the obvious sincerity and goodwill of the whistleblowers. Macchiarini comes across like a mysterious celebrity permitting his fans a rare glimpse behind the scenes. But the whistleblowers—Matthias Corbascio, Kalle Grinnemo, and Thomas Fux—seem so earnest and alarmed that they are virtually impossible to dismiss. (A fourth whistleblower, Oscar Simonson, does not appear in the film.)

Whether the outcome should be counted as a success is unclear. While Macchiarini was finally convicted of assault and sentenced to prison in June 2023, none of the whistleblowers admit to any confidence that the Karolinska Institute has learned anything from the scandal. Yet much of what they achieved can be attributed to a conscious decision they made at the outset of their struggle: that they would work together in solidarity as a group.

• • •

Macchiarini's dramatic rise began in 2008 when he performed a novel surgical procedure on Claudia Castillo, a young mother of two in Barcelona whose trachea had collapsed after a tuberculosis infection. Macchiarini took a trachea from a deceased donor, stripped it down to its cartilaginous structure, and seeded it with stem cells taken from Castillo's bone marrow. The theory was that Castillo's stem cells would attach themselves to the cadaveric trachea and transform into tracheal cells, making the trachea functional and eliminating the need for the immunosuppressant drugs that are necessary after transplants. A "milestone in medicine," CNN proclaimed.[2] Two years and several transplants later, Macchiarini got an offer to move to the Karolinska Institute.

"He was a very powerful and colorful person in many ways," says Dr. Karl-Henrik (Kalle) Grinnemo in *The Experiments*. "Your chin just dropped, and you just stood and absorbed it all and thought: 'What an amazing person we have here!'" Grinnemo and Dr. Matthias Corbascio, both cardiothoracic surgeons at the Karolinska, were asked to help Macchiarini set up a new transplantation unit. By that point, however, some of the earlier transplant patients were beginning to have problems, including Claudia Castillo, whose transplanted trachea had collapsed. So Macchiarini proposed to begin doing another kind of procedure. Instead of transplanting cadaveric tracheas, he would use a synthetic trachea made of plastic.

The idea was audacious. Using scans of a patient's trachea, scientists would build a synthetic scaffold—a replica of the trachea—out of polymerized plastic. Macchiarini's team would place the scaffold in a "bioreactor" (a small rectangular container roughly the size of a shoebox) filled with a solution of stem cells harvested from the patient's bone marrow. There the scaffold would be rotated slowly like a rotisserie chicken until it was seeded by stem cells. When the seeded scaffold was implanted in the patient, the stem cells would send out chemical signals for the patient's bone marrow to send more stem cells. Over time the synthetic trachea would gradually be transformed into something like a natural part of the patient's body.

Macchiarini identified his first experimental subject in the spring of 2011. Andemariam Beyene was an Etritrean graduate student in his late thirties. Married with two young children, Beyene was studying geothermal energy in Iceland. Photos show a handsome young man with a shy smile and a pencil mustache, like that of Nick Charles in *The Thin Man*. Two years earlier, Beyene had started to have trouble breathing. Doctors found a tumor the size of a golf ball growing into his trachea. He was treated with surgery and radiation, but his condition continued to worsen. According to Macchiarini, doctors at Harvard had seen Beyene and given him less than six months to live.

When Macchiarini implanted the synthetic trachea in June of 2011, he invited Kalle Grinnemo to participate. The invitation felt like an honor. "It was almost like being in a bubble when you were in there. You didn't even hear what people said because you were so focused," Grinnemo says in *The Experiments*. The procedure took twelve hours. "And when it was all over, we were all on a high. You were both tired and happy, and of course hungry. I remember we all got in a car and drove off to Max and bought hamburgers for everybody. And just sat and stuffed our faces and celebrated that it had gone so well." Grinnemo calls it a "hallelujah moment." He says, "We all felt we had made history."

A month later, when Beyene was discharged from the hospital, international media outlets reported the procedure as a groundbreaking medical first. "It's working like a normal windpipe," Macchiarini told National Public Radio. "He's able to cough. He's able to expel his secretions. He's breathing normally. He has the sensation he's breathing."[3] Macchiarini announced plans to perform his synthetic implants in the United States, including one in a child who was born without a trachea. In late November 2011, Macchiarini and his colleagues published their results in *The Lancet*, one of the world's most respected medical journals.[4]

Yet there were early indications that not everything was as it seemed. After the apparent success of the operation on Beyene, surgeons at University College London tried implanting a synthetic trachea in Keziah Shorten, a nineteen-year-old woman into whom Macchiarini had transplanted a cadaveric trachea, which had eventually failed. Shorten died several months later.[5] In November 2011, Macchiarini implanted his second synthetic trachea in Christopher Lyles, a thirty-year-old electrical engineer from Maryland with tracheal cancer. "He went home in very good shape," Macchiarini told the *New York Times*.[6] Lyles lived only five months.

The bluntest critic of the procedure was Dr. Pierre Delaere, a professor of respiratory surgery at Katholieke Universiteit (KU) Leuven, in Belgium. According to Delaere, there was no scientific research to suggest that a synthetic trachea would work. "You don't have to be a doctor to know that a synthetic trachea cannot transform into a living trachea by applying bone marrow on it," he says. Delaere felt that it was only a matter of time before the patients died. "If I had the option of a synthetic trachea or a firing squad," he says, "I'd choose the last option because it would be the least painful form of execution." Delaere tried repeatedly to alert authorities at the Karolinska Institute of the dangers to their patients, but his warnings were dismissed.[7]

Macchiarini played the part of swashbuckling surgical hero as if he were born to the role. "I'm just a surgeon, I need action," Macchiarini said in an adulatory profile by *The Lancet* in 2012. "I'm like a wild animal that does not need to be in a cage, I need to express my convictions that I can help a patient with innovative things."[8] Macchiarini called himself a "citizen of the world"—born in Switzerland of Italian parents in 1958; medical school at the University of Pisa, in Italy; a fellowship in thoracic surgery at the University of Alabama-Birmingham; and, most importantly, ten years at the Centre Chirurgical Marie-Lannelongue, in Paris. "This was the turning point of my life," Macchiarini said of his time in Paris, the point at which he was transformed into a "cutting edge" thoracic surgeon. He predicted a revolution in transplant medicine, a future where replacement organs would be grown in labs and immunosuppressant drugs would be a thing of the past.

A Leap of Faith, NBC's 2014 documentary, reinforced

Macchiarini's celebrity status, comparing his accomplishments to Neil Armstrong's walk on the moon. American surgeons vouched for his brilliance. The families of his patients expressed their humble gratitude. To the critics who said he was moving too quickly with such novel surgical procedures, Macchiarini replied, "As a surgeon you're a risk-taker, especially if you do these crazy things."[9] When Macchiarini wasn't saving lives in the operating room, he was speeding around on his motorcycle in a leather jacket and aviator sunglasses.

Oscar Simonson, one of the surgeons who would later blow the whistle, remembers traveling to the Mayo Clinic for a conference where Macchiarini was giving a keynote address. "He was like the second coming of the Messiah," Simonson says. Macchiarini spoke to the group about "brain scaffolds." His idea was to translate his stem cell technology into a treatment for patients who had sustained frontal lobe damage, such as American soldiers injured in war. "Everybody was applauding this, of course, but that made absolutely no sense, actually," Simonson says.

After operating on Beyene and Lyles, Macchiarini performed two more synthetic trachea implants in Russia, neither of which would end well. But it was a spectacularly ill-fated transplant at the Karolinska Institute on a young Turkish woman, Yesim Cetir, that set off the chain of events leading to his downfall.

• • •

Like almost every surgeon I know, Kalle Grinnemo walks very fast. He is leading me through the streets of central Stockholm, and I have no real idea where we are. We are looking for a place to have lunch. As I trail behind him with my overstuffed backpack, sweating moderately, I am fighting the urge to trot. It is a warm, sunny day in early August of 2021, and I have just gotten to the city from Arlanda Airport. As we pass the Stockholm Concert Hall, Grinnemo points out that this is where the Nobel Prizes are presented. "Somehow I can't look at those prizes in the same way now," I tell him. "Me neither," Grinnemo replies. Soon he identifies a suitable restaurant, and we settle in for a lunch of poached coalfish and potatoes, with my backpack occupying the next chair.

Grinnemo has a kind face and a thoughtful, understated manner. He wears rectangular black glasses, and there is a touch of gray in his close-cropped hair. Although Grinnemo left the Karolinska Institute several years ago for a position at Uppsala University, the wounds from his experience at the Karolinska are still evident when he speaks. He knew Macchiarini better than any of the other whistleblowers, and he was the first to feel the heat when they began to speak out. "I was sort of closest to the fire," Grinnemo says. When Yesim Cetir arrived in 2012, the blaze intensified.

Cetir was a university student in Turkey who came to the Karolinska Institute after a botched surgical procedure. During an elective operation to prevent excessive hand sweating, surgeons in Turkey had nicked Cetir's trachea. The injury was not life-threatening, but Cetir was left with a chronic cough and a drainage tube in her chest.[10] She lived at home and planned to become a teacher. Photos of her at the time show a pretty, dark-haired young woman who looks like a teenaged girl.

When Cetir was admitted to the hospital, Macchiarini made the unusual decision to perform an exploratory thoracotomy. Instead of simply doing more imaging studies, he opened up Cetir's chest to see what damage had been done to her trachea. The procedure was a fiasco. As Macchiarini was putting traction on the trachea to visualize the injury, the wall of the trachea burst. There was a massive air leakage, and the right lung started to bleed uncontrollably. Macchiarini had to remove the right lung in order to get air into the left one. "It was sort of a panic situation in the OR," Grinnemo says. "Paolo just ripped out the right lung, basically." To keep Cetir from dying, Macchiarini was forced to put her on ECMO (extracorporeal membrane oxygenation), a device similar to a heart-lung bypass machine.

Because her condition was so dire, Macchiarini implanted Cetir with a synthetic trachea two weeks later. Initially, the synthetic trachea seemed to work well. She was taken off ECMO. But the day after her surgery, Cetir crashed. Alarms sounded on the ward. Grinnemo rushed into the room to see Cetir, her eyes wide and terrified, waving her arms as if she was trying to get something out of her throat. Her oxygen levels had dropped precipitously. She needed CPR, but the presence of a probe in her esophagus meant that chest compressions might damage her trachea. Grinnemo and his colleague, Matthias Corbascio, did compressions anyway. When Cetir didn't respond, they put her back on ECMO and stabilized her. Afterward, Grinnemo and Corbascio just stared at each other and asked, "How did this happen?"[11]

Although Cetir was eventually weaned from ECMO, she remained in fragile condition in the intensive care unit for months. Her airway had to be suctioned every four hours to prevent her from suffocating, and she required a feeding tube for nutrition. A second synthetic implant in 2013 did not help. The medical attention Cetir required was unrelenting, and the responsibility largely fell on Thomas Fux, an intensive care specialist. When the other whistleblowers speak of Fux and the perseverance he brought to the care of Cetir, it is with a kind of hushed reverence. "He almost moved into the hospital for three years," Grinnemo says. "He really dedicated his whole life actually during that period for her in order to keep her alive, and so he did an enormous job."

Grinnemo and Corbascio began to wonder about Andemariam Beyene, Macchiarini's first synthetic trachea patient. Beyene had returned to Iceland, and they assumed he was still doing well. But Corbascio remembers running into an ear, nose, and throat specialist in the changing room of his department and asking how things were going with Beyene. "And he said, 'It's going straight to hell,'" Corbascio says. "And I was like, what? That was news." Beyene's graft was infected, obstructed, and leaking. In January 2014, Beyene died. Fux insisted on an autopsy and attended it as an observer. The autopsy showed that the synthetic trachea had never healed. It was loose, degraded, and almost totally disconnected from the surrounding tissue.[12] At that point Grinnemo says that he and the others began to ask, "What kind of science is behind the use of these synthetic grafts?"

A disturbing clue came from Oscar Simonson, a cardio-thoracic surgeon with experience doing scientific work with animal models. To see how the angiogenesis and reepithelial-ization of the synthetic grafts worked, Simonson began to col-laborate on rat experiments with Macchiarini's postdoctoral fellow, a surgeon from Germany named Phillip Jungebluth. Simonson came back to Macchiarini with bad news. The syn-thetic grafts caused an enormous inflammatory response in rats. This was not the response Macchiarini wanted to hear. He responded by ejecting Simonson from the team. "He hated criticism," Grinnemo says. "So, if you brought up something which was against the way he was thinking, you were immedi-ately kicked out."

Up until that point, Grinnemo and the others had assumed that Macchiarini had thoroughly tested the synthetic tracheas in rats and pigs before implanting one in a human being. Mat-thias Corbascio can remember the exact moment when he realized this wasn't true. He says, "There was a group of vis-iting scientists from the United States, and Macchiarini was giving a lecture about his research, and he showed data of pigs where he had implanted a decellularized trachea, a decellu-larized windpipe. And then he jumped from that to showing plastic windpipes in people." If Macchiarini had implanted the plastic windpipes in the pigs, and not merely decellularized windpipes, he would have shown that data. "And that's when I realized, oh my God, this guy hasn't tested this in an animal," Corbascio says. "I still remember what I was wearing. That realization just made the hair on my body stand up. You know, I got goosebumps on my whole body."

Relations with Macchiarini had begun to break down. Not only did Macchiarini refuse to take any responsibility for the problems facing Cetir, but he had also continued full steam ahead with synthetic implants on patients in Russia. At a meeting in the fall of 2013, Grinnemo asked Macchiarini about the complications they were seeing. Macchiarini lost his temper and threatened to make life miserable for Grinnemo. Shortly afterward, Macchiarini and Phillip Jungebluth filed a complaint accusing Grinnemo of stealing research data. Grinnemo says, "And then we started to understand, okay, so this is the way he will start to act. He will discredit the four of us in different ways."

The group of four whistleblowers came together gradually. Kalle Grinnemo and Matthias Corbascio were old friends; they knew each other's families and took vacations together. Corbascio had also co-supervised Grinnemo's doctoral dissertation. Oscar Simonson knew Grinnemo because their heart research was in similar areas. The only member of the group who was not a cardiovascular surgeon was Thomas Fux, the intensive care specialist who began taking care of Yesim Cetir. But Corbascio and Fux knew each other well from their clinical work in the hospital. "Thomas would take care of the most complex patients in the ICU," Corbascio tells me. "We got to know him that way, discussing and taking care of these very sick patients."

The group of four decided they had to save Cetir. They started going through all the medical records. Corbascio remembers that at one point, they were sitting together in his office talking about Macchiarini when Simonson said, "I wonder if this guy has actually got ethical permission to do this stuff," adding, "I bet he doesn't." Corbascio was skeptical. "No, come on, that's just ridiculous," he said. "That's insane." But they wrote to the Central Ethical Review Board, the committee responsible for overseeing medical research, and sure enough, Macchiarini did not have permission.[13] Corbascio says, "We were laughing and horrified at the same time. I mean, what the hell is going on?" It was unfathomable that anyone would start these experiments without the proper regulatory approval. Corbascio says, "You can't even imagine it as a scientist, as a doctor."

The four whistleblowers spent the summer of 2014 combing through scientific reports and patient records. By August they were ready to submit a massive, thoroughly detailed report to Anders Hamsten, the vice-chancellor of the Karolinska Institute.[14] They knew that their report would not be welcomed. Corbascio insisted that they all join the doctors' union for protection. Grinnemo joked that they should pack the report in diapers because Hamsten would shit himself when he read it. Yet months passed and they did not even receive an acknowledgment.

• • •

In early August, when the days are still long and the sun sits low in the sky, Stockholm feels like an enchanted city. Located on an archipelago where Lake Mälaren flows into the Baltic Sea, the city encompasses fourteen islands connected by bridges. You can wander the streets for miles and never stray far from the water. At the heart of the city is the *Gamla stan*, the old town, with its winding cobblestone streets, medieval stone churches, and right in its main square, the Nobel Prize Museum. Housed in an imposing, yellow, eighteenth-century building, the museum was opened in 2001 to celebrate the one-hundredth anniversary of the Nobel Prize. It is intended to be a "reflecting and forward-looking and spirited memory of Nobel laureates and their achievements, as well as of the Nobel Prize and Alfred Nobel."

In his will, Alfred Nobel specified the Karolinska Institute, a former training facility for military surgeons, as the home of the Nobel Prize for Physiology or Medicine. The main campus is in the suburb of Solna, just north of the city. But neither Solna nor the campus of the Karolinska Institute have any of Stockholm's charm. A bus stop sits in front of one of the main Karolinska Hospital buildings, a red-brick, utilitarian structure with rows of small rectangular windows on each floor. The small academic campus has few of the traditional signifiers that are customary on American or British university campuses. There is no quadrangle, no bell tower, no Victorian spires or chapels. What stands out are the corporate logos on a couple of buildings and a street named Nobels Vag. In August, the most visible human presence is an occasional maintenance worker with a shovel or a weed eater, taking care of the lawn.

Oscar Simsonson believes that the Nobel Prize has been a curse for the Karolinska Institute. "Since we hand out the Nobel Prize, it's a big problem because people start thinking that they are that gifted, or they *are* the Nobel Prize," he tells me. Of the four whistleblowers, Simonson is the only one who trained at the Karolinska Institute from medical school onward. He compares it to joining a cult. So important is the selection of the Nobel Prize, Simsonson says, that faculty members at the Karolinska Institute would rather be on the committee that awards the prize than to receive a Nobel Prize itself. "This is sort of the Holy Ghost of the Karolinska. It's this thing with the Nobel, where nothing else really matters," he says. "Your goal is to come into this Nobel Committee. I mean, that's your single goal of life."

Simonson and I are drinking beer at a table outside Rolfs Kök in Stockholm. He is a big, cheerful man in a white baseball cap who walks even faster than Kalle Grinnemo. We have just finished a delicious dinner of "witch," a fish previously unfamiliar to me, as well as potato pancakes with Swedish roe, which Simonson insists are far superior to American roe. Like Grinnemo, Simonson has moved from the Karolinska to the University of Uppsala, but he and his family still have their apartment in Stockholm. Simonson is funny, blunt, and full of energy, even though he has spent all day in the operating room. Although he describes himself as the skeptic in the group, he strikes me as the most upbeat and optimistic. Simonson tells me he lived in Minneapolis for a year when he was a child. Among his memories of Minnesota are a Montessori school, a friend with pinball machines and video games in his basement, and a trip to Disney World, where he was too little to ride on the Space Mountain roller coaster.

"The Karolinska has never been a university," Simonson says. "It only has medicine." Unlike most traditional universities, the Karolinska Institute does not have faculties of law, literature, mathematics, or other disciplines. "It's more like a research hotel," he says. "It's much more labeling and you know, PR, than a normal university." When he was a medical student, Simonson says, criticism of the Karolinska was forbidden. It simply wasn't allowed. While Simonson concedes that doctors are an unusually obedient and conformist group, he believes that the doctors at the Karolinska Institute have taken these traits to an extreme. "I think it still is kind of unique in that aspect," he says. "You could probably find other crazy places like that, but it's to a level that is, you know, not only not healthy, but it's really abnormal."

Simonson says he wasn't surprised by the behavior of the

Karolinska leaders when the evidence of Macchiarini's fraud and negligence emerged. He never expected any of them to do the right thing. "I never had that illusion," he says. "I've seen too much, and you know, I was brought up in this kind of environment." Simonson said he went into the fight with certain baseline assumptions about how the Karolinska authorities would respond, none of them good. "The assumption is that the Karolinska will always try to lie, because it always does that," he says. Another of his assumptions was that the authorities would retaliate.

After the whistleblowers submitted their report and got no response, they spent nearly a year and a half trying to stop Macchiarini. They alerted regulatory bodies, funding authorities, and the press. Nothing worked. "The Central Ethical Review Board didn't want to touch this thing. They sent a two-sentence letter to me saying that 'Well, this isn't research; this is medical care,'" Matthias Corbascio says. "Everything we tried failed, basically. I mean, we were just losing our minds." They were not alone in their frustration. In June 2014, Pierre Delaere, in Leuven, filed a complaint of scientific conduct against Macchiarini, but the Ethics Council for the Karolinska Institute dismissed Delaere's concerns, saying that they were of a "philosophy-of-science kind rather than of a research-ethical kind."[15] In June 2015, the Swedish Research Council suspended Macchiarini's funding; five months later, the Karolinska Institute appointed him for another year.[16]

One incident illustrates just how determined the leaders of the Karolinska Institute were to protect Macchiarini. In November of 2014, a leaked copy of the whistleblowers' report came into the hands of the *New York Times*, which published an article titled "Leading Surgeon Is Accused of Misconduct in Experimental Transplant Operations."[17] The article detailed several of the most serious allegations against Macchiarini: that he had never obtained ethical permission to conduct his experiments, that his 2011 study in *The Lancet* had misrepresented the outcome of Beyene's implant, and that of the three patients at the Karolinska Institute that Macchiarini had given synthetic implants, only Beyene had signed a consent form—and the form was dated two weeks *after* his surgery. The publicity generated by the article all but forced the Karolinska Institute to act. Anders Hamsten, the vice-chancellor, said he would ask for an external inquiry.

Retaliation against the whistleblowers came quickly. According to Simonson, the whistleblowers were told that they had violated patient privacy and would be fired immediately. That didn't happen, but in December the Karolinska Institute informed the whistleblowers that the head of the cardiothoracic clinic would deliver a formal warning, the last step before an employee is terminated.[18] The Karolinska Institute also reported the whistleblowers to the police. "I was called down to the police and put in a room with no windows, with a tape recorder and a lawyer and a policeman in front of me, and interrogated. That was pretty scary," Corbascio says. "It was exactly what it's like on television. And you know, it's hard to be a tough guy in that room." The accusations were baseless; the whistleblowers had anonymized all the identities in their report, and Corbascio had applied in advance for ethical permission to access patient records. "I wrote that ethics application because I knew that they were going to try to fire us," he says.

In the spring of 2015, the external inquiry Hamsten had promised was completed. Dr. Bengt Gerdin, an emeritus professor at Uppsala University Hospital, concluded that Macchiarini was guilty of scientific misconduct.[19] The inquiry didn't address any potential abuses of human subjects, but the result of the inquiry was clear. Macchiarini had falsified his research.

But even an external corroboration of misconduct didn't

deter the Karolinska Institute leaders. It took months for them to respond, and when they finally came to a conclusion, they called a press conference. "We asked if we could attend the press conference, and they said no," Simonson says. "They then called our boss at the time and said that they were hiring guards to stop us from attending." Accompanied by members of the Nobel Committee, vice-chancellor Anders Hamsten disavowed Gerdin's external inquiry and proclaimed his confidence in Macchiarini. The whistleblowers were stunned. Macchiarini responded with gratitude. "To have been falsely accused of such serious misconduct is every researcher's nightmare," he said.[20] *The Lancet* applauded the decision with an editorial titled "Paolo Macchiarini Is Not Guilty of Scientific Misconduct."[21]

Grinnemo remembers this entire period as a very dark time. The stress was overwhelming. "I mean, I couldn't sleep. I was always thinking of this next strategic move," he says. People he considered friends stopped returning his calls and emails. He could not concentrate on his research. He found it hard to give his children the attention they needed. "It was also hard doing surgery, to be standing there focusing on the operation," he says. The thought that he might have sacrificed his career for a futile cause sent him into a panic. Corbascio felt the same way. The hostility at work was palpable. He says, "I think that Kalle and I were like the two most hated people at Karolinska, and I've no doubt about that."

When the whistleblowers learned that Bosse Lindquist was working on a documentary about Macchiarini for Swedish Television, they didn't consider it good news. "We didn't know if we were going to laugh or cry," Grinnemo says. They assumed that Lindquist, like most other journalists, was planning to give Macchiarini the star treatment. So when Lindquist asked to interview them, they said no. But Lindquist kept pressing. He said, "Honestly, what kind of choice do you have?

What is your situation like now?" After considering that question, Grinnemo says, they decided that, well, yes, their current situation sucked. Reluctantly they agreed to cooperate, but it was an act of faith and desperation. They had no idea what story the documentary would tell.

· · ·

If there is an archetypal whistleblowing story, a script that fixed the pattern for the whistleblowing stories that would come later, it is Henrik Ibsen's 1882 play, *An Enemy of the People*. In the play, Thomas Stockmann is a doctor in a Norwegian spa town who begins seeing an abnormally high number of patients with typhoid and other illnesses. Suspecting that the baths are poisoned, Stockmann discovers that a tannery is oozing toxins into the water. Alarmed, yet also elated that he has identified the problem, Stockmann assumes he'll be celebrated for saving innocent lives. He plans to be humble about it, of course. He would never accept an award or a raise. "I have done nothing more than my duty," Stockmann says. "It is a splendid thing for a man to be able to feel that he has done a service to his native town and to his fellow-citizens."[22] Applauded by his family, Stockmann happily twirls his wife around the kitchen.

Of course, the last thing anyone wants to hear is that the economic engine of the town is poisoning people. So Stockmann is vilified for his discovery, not celebrated. His friends turn on him. His brother, the mayor, threatens him. The newspaper reporters he thought were allies turn out to be scoundrels and invertebrates. Feeling threatened, Stockmann becomes obstinate. His humility turns to arrogance. When the atmosphere gets ugly at a town meeting, Stockmann lectures the crowd on its stupidity. He compares the town to a dog kennel, implying that he is one of the purebreds. "Do you not think the poodle's brain is developed to quite a different degree than the cur?" he asks them. "There is a tremendous difference between poodle-men and cur-men."[23]

The more heated the argument gets, the more Stockmann sounds like a fascist. "All who live by lies ought to be exterminated like vermin!" he shouts. "Let the whole country perish, let all these people be exterminated."[24] The meeting ends with the angry crowd shouting that Stockmann is an enemy of the people. The next day Stockmann is fired from his job. So is his daughter. His wealthy father-in-law turns on him. But still he refuses to give in. The play ends with a defiant Stockmann uttering the play's most famous line: "The strongest man in the world is he who stands most alone."[25]

As it was in nineteenth-century Norway, so it was in twenty-first-century Sweden—at least to some extent. Many of the plot points in *An Enemy of the People* were repeated in the Macchiarini scandal: the attacks on idealistic whistleblowers, the duplicity of institutional authorities, the circling of the wagons in response to an economic threat. Macchiarini's synthetic tracheas were to the Karolinska Institute what the baths were to Stockmann's town; no one wanted to hear that they were based on fraud. Even outsiders couldn't imagine that the whistleblowers were telling the truth. "In Sweden we are brought up with the sense that we don't have any corruption in the country," Simonson says. A cover-up was especially hard to imagine at the Karolinska Institute, given the respect it commands in Sweden. "Many people were simply unwilling to consider the idea that this university could ever do something as stupid and diabolical as this," Corbascio says. "It's just unfathomable for a Swede."

An Enemy of the People has enjoyed a revival of interest in recent years, thanks in part to Donald Trump's use of the phrase "enemies of the people" to refer to the press. Yet the fit with current events has always been a little uncomfortable. The newspaper reporters in *An Enemy of the People* are not heroic figures speaking truth to power. They are self-serving cowards. And while Stockmann is right about the poisoned water, it is hard to listen to his fiery eugenicist tirade about "poodle men" without laughing. He sounds like a cross between Adolf Hitler and Fred Willard's clueless color commentator in *Best in Show*. It is no wonder that many contemporary adaptations of the play either soften his speech or leave it out entirely.

Even more disorienting is Stockmann's final declaration. Throughout the battle over the poisoned baths, Stockmann has been supported by a close circle of intimates. His family has stood by him. His daughter has sacrificed her job for the cause. When Stockmann and his family are evicted from their home, one of their closest friends offers them his house. Yet Stockmann proclaims that he is strong because he stands completely alone. For Stockmann to believe this demands a certain degree of self-deception, but even if he were right, it seems like an odd moral aspiration. Stockmann doesn't declare that he stands for truth or justice. He doesn't proclaim that he will spare nothing to save innocent lives. Instead, like a figure conjured by Nietzsche, he points his finger in the air and proclaims his solitary moral strength.

That *An Enemy of the People* has become such an emblematic Scandinavian play carries a certain irony. Greta Thunberg aside, the Scandinavian countries are not famous for their rebels, dissenters, and renegades. They are known for their collectivist ethic, their generous systems of social welfare, and their culture of political consensus. The Danish-Norwegian novelist Aksel Sandemose satirized the Scandinavian obsession with social conformity in his 1933 novel *En flyktning krysser sitt spor* (*A Fugitive Crosses his Tracks*), which is set in a fictional small town called Jante. Sandemose laid out ten rules of social behavior in Jante, such as "You're not to think *you* can teach *us* anything" and "You're not to think *you* know more than *we* do." In Scandinavian countries, the phrase *jan-teloven*, or "law of Jante," serves as shorthand for an attitude of disapproval toward individuality, ostentation, and personal ambition. To stand out from the crowd is strongly discouraged; to boast about your moral and genetic superiority is unthinkable.

A possible explanation comes from Henrik Berggren and Lars Trägårdh in their book *The Swedish Theory of Love*. Berggren and Trägårdh explain that the Swedish collectivist ethic is compatible with a particular kind of individualism. Collectivism doesn't mean that Swedes are an especially sociable people, like the Italians. Just the opposite: immigrants to Sweden are often struck by the Swedes' emotional independence and need for solitude. In Sweden, individualism translates to freedom from social dependency on intimates. Berggren and Trägårdh write, "For Swedes, the ideal state is a Crusoe-like existence in nature, living as an autonomous individual."[26] People who must rely on other people for kindness or charity are seen as inauthentic and untrustworthy. Hence the moral logic of the generous, collectivist Swedish state: it maximizes the independence of individuals by liberating them from the kindness of their friends and family. This is what Berggren and Trägårdh mean by "the Swedish theory of love."

What binds Swedes together is not sociability so much as a high degree of social trust. Swedes trust one another, they trust the government, and they trust Swedish authorities. It is partly for this reason that Swedish society functions as well as it does. As the journalist Andrew Brown writes, "Swedes know how they should behave, and they expect everyone else to behave in the same way."[27] Social conformity keeps the wheels of Swedish society greased and frictionless. Everyone can trust that others feel as obligated as they do to stick to the rules. On the other hand, of course, this leaves them vulnerable to exploitation by people who don't feel the same sense of obligation, such as Paolo Macchiarini.

Unlike Thomas Stockmann, none of the Karolinska whistleblowers had any illusions of standing alone. They knew that was a recipe for failure. Their decision to work together as a team was carefully planned. "It's like flying to the moon," Simonson says. "If you're going to do that, you need the right people." All their decisions were collaborative. When any member of the group met individually with someone at the Karolinska Institute, that person taped the conversation so that the rest could hear what was said. Grinnemo says, "We said from the very beginning that if we were going to succeed with this mission to stop Macchiarini, and stop this implantation, we need to agree on every move we make."

Grinnemo says that each of them felt discouraged at various times in their struggle, but others were always there to help. "During the beginning I was the one who was really down, because they went really, really hard on me. So, I was down for the count. And then the others helped me out," he says. At other times, three of the four were demoralized and there was only one insisting they would get through it together. Grinnemo says, "If it had been only me that was filing these complaints, then I would never have succeeded, never ever."

Although Thomas Stockmann is a flawed hero with a confused message, there is something familiar about his moral determination—the way he responds to a hostile crowd not by softening his principles but by obstinately refusing to back down. This ethical obstinacy is a trait that many whistleblowers share. Matthias Corbascio pointed me to a Swedish word, *rättspatos*, for which there is no good English translation. The word *rätts* is usually translated as "justice," and *patos* as "pathos," from the Greek word for suffering. But *rättspatos*, according to Corbascio, is "a pathological feeling of what's right." For a person with a strong *rättspatos*, there is simply no choice but to speak out against injustice. He compares *rättspatos* to what Martin Luther King Jr called "a vocation of agony." He says, "It's sort of a quality that, you know, if something is wrong, then come hell or high water, it's wrong. In the end you're just going to go to the mattresses if need be." He pauses. "Stubbornness, I guess."

• • •

Bosse Lindquist remembers when he was approached about making a documentary on Paolo Macchiarini. "I was actually thinking of resigning," he says. Lindquist had not been happy with his recent work. His bosses at Swedish Television seemed to want sensational films that would attract a big audience, while he was interested in subtler, more complicated stories. When his boss showed him the accusations that the Karolinska whistleblowers had made, his first instinct was to say no. He had such tremendous respect for the Karolinska Institute. The researchers at the Karolinska that Lindquist knew personally were all honest, conscientious scientists, and the accusations against Macchiarini seemed far-fetched. But after a few days, Lindquist decided that the story would be interesting even if the accusations were untrue. Why would four doctors at the Karolinska Institute make such bizarre claims? He made an appointment to speak with Matthias Corbascio.

When Lindquist knocked on the door at Corbascio's apartment, it was answered by a tall, bald American with fierce eyes and a Black Sabbath T-shirt. For two hours Corbascio ranted about Macchiarini's crimes, comparing Macchiarini to Josef Mengele at Auschwitz. "I thought he was probably crazy," Lindquist says. "He was at a breaking point." At that time Lindquist didn't yet appreciate how panicked a whistleblower can get when his warnings have been completely ignored. What kept him from dismissing Corbascio's testimony as the ravings of a deranged man was the arrival of Corbascio's wife, a calm, Swedish cancer researcher who seemed eminently sensible and clear-headed. "Is all this true?" Lindquist asked her. Yes, she nodded, it's all true. There was a quiet desperation in her eyes. "She was on a sinking ship," he says. "She looked at me as if I was the last hand stretching at a sinking ship."

Lindquist and I are drinking coffee on the balcony of his apartment in the Södermalm district of Stockholm. We first met in the fall of 2018, when I invited him to screen *The Experiments* at the University of Minnesota and speak about the Macchiarini scandal. He brought his son, Hugo, along for the trip, and we became friends. Lindquist is a modest, soft-spoken man in his sixties with a dry sense of humor, a philosophical cast of mind, and a deep curiosity about the world. Whenever I call or email him to talk, the response is as likely to come back from Tanzania, Italy, or Thailand as it is from Stockholm.

Lindquist and his crew spent nearly twelve months following Macchiarini and digging deeper into the accusations against him. It took a month or two before Lindquist began to give any credence to the whistleblowers' warnings. Macchiarini had a grand vision about the future of transplant medicine and he was very convincing. "I liked him, actually," Lindquist says. Con artists are often described as charming and charismatic, but Lindquist says Macchiarini had something different—a certain vulnerability, even boyishness. Lindquist found it touching. Not until the summer of 2015 did the balance of evidence finally begin to tip against Macchiarini. By the time the first episode of the three-part documentary appeared on Swedish Television in January 2016, the case against Macchiarini was airtight.

The stage for the documentary was set by an article published in early January 2016, only two weeks before *The Experiments* aired. Writing in *Vanity Fair*, the journalist Adam Ciralsky laid out a brazen story of intrigue and deception in Macchiarini's personal life.[28] A year and a half earlier,

NBC News had profiled Macchiarini in a fawning, Emmy-nominated special called *A Leap of Faith*. During the production Macchiarini had become romantically involved with Benita Alexander, an NBC producer, to whom he soon proposed. By that point, Macchiarini was such a celebrity that it didn't seem far-fetched when he began to announce elaborate wedding plans. According to *Vanity Fair*, he told Alexander that the ceremony would take place at the Apostolic Palace of Castel Gandolfo, where Pope Francis would officiate. Andrea Bocelli would sing. Guests would include Vladimir Putin, Russell Crowe, Elton John, John Legend, and Kenny Rogers—not to mention the Obamas, the Sarkozys, and the Clintons. Macchiarini and Alexander sent out engraved wedding invitations sheathed in lambskin.

Two months before the wedding, Alexander got an email from a friend with the subject line "The Pope." It linked to an article stating that Pope Francis would be in South America at the same time as the wedding. With that, the charade fell apart. Aided by a private investigator, Alexander learned that virtually every detail Macchiarini had provided about the wedding was false. The pope had no idea who Macchiarini was. Andrea Bocelli would not be performing. According to a public records search, Macchiarini was still married to his wife of nearly thirty years and living with another woman. Further investigation suggested that he had fabricated several items on his curriculum vitae, claiming degrees he did not have and positions he had never held. Piece by piece, the elaborate story that Macchiarini had told Alexander fell apart.

Two weeks later, the first episode of *The Experiments* aired. "I remember it very clearly," Grinnemo says. "Everyone was sitting at home, the whole family around, watching that documentary, and we were sitting with the phones, actually, to call each other if, shit, this is not good." There had been other documentaries and news stories about Macchiarini, of course, and they generally portrayed him as a hero. But as *The Experiments* progressed, Grinnemo says, the realization began to sink in: "Oh my God, he nailed him. He understood the situation. This is fantastic." But along with that happy realization came another one: "Oh, my God. This will not be fun to come back to work right now."

The Experiments unfolds with the narrative drama of a crime movie. "Is he a genius, or is he a fraud?" Lindquist asks in the introduction. Macchiarini has the full support of the Karolinska Institute, yet his patients all seem to be dying. Lindquist proceeds to expose Macchiarini's lies simply by showing the visual evidence: video footage from bronchoscopies, firsthand testimony from the whistleblowers, conversations filmed as they occurred in clinics and hospital rooms. When the family members of the victims speak to Lindquist, the pain in their voices sounds raw and exposed.

Much of the action in *The Experiments* takes place not at the Karolinska Institute, but in Russia. After Macchiarini implanted the synthetic trachea in cancer patients, he decided to try it as an elective procedure in patients who were in relatively good health. This was an astonishing choice. The procedure had never even been tested in animals. Yet Russian authorities gave him permission to start a formal clinical trial in Russia. Casting around for potential candidates, Macchiarini and his team invited people to send videos explaining why they should be chosen, like applicants for a reality television show. The winner was Julia Tuulik, a young teacher and former dancer in St. Petersburg. Although she was healthy, a car accident had left her with a tracheostomy, and in order to speak, she had to cover the opening with her hand. She hoped the surgery would let her sing to her son. Accompanied by a German film crew, Macchiarini gave Tuulik a synthetic trachea in June 2012 at Kuban State University, in Krasnodar, Russia. A few days later, the two appeared together at a triumphant press conference.

Tuulik's condition began to deteriorate shortly after the procedure. "She had bouts of coughing, lasting for hours, and she could barely breathe," her husband says in *The Experiments*. Macchiarini replaced the synthetic trachea with a second one, but it didn't work either. "It smelled of rotting flesh," Tuulik's mother says. Tuulik lived for less than two and a half years.

As Lindquist investigated Tuulik's death, he obtained access to unedited film footage from a German production crew that had profiled Macchiarini. One scene showed Macchiarini in the spring of 2012, shortly after the death of Christopher Lyles, walking on a beach and speaking on his cell phone with David Green, of Harvard Biosciences, the manufacturer of a "bioreactor" used to grow stem cells for the synthetic trachea. Macchiarini confesses that the synthetic tracheas are faulty. "Listen, what happens is that the [trachea] scaffolds dry out," Macchiarini says. Yet only a few weeks later, he will implant that same kind of faulty synthetic trachea in Tuulik.

A second conversation is even more alarming. Macchiarini has just arrived at the Kuban State Medical University when he is approached by a thoracic surgeon wearing blue scrubs who asks, "Do you know about the problem?" All three of the available synthetic tracheas are defective, the surgeon explains. One is too short, another has holes, and a third is unstable. Yet Macchiarini barely hesitates. Rather than postponing the surgery, he decides to proceed with the short trachea without telling Tuulik. "We know this material is very safe," David Green tells Tuulik as she perches on the side of her bed. "You're in very good hands. . . . Paolo is the best surgeon in the world." "I know," Tuulik replies, nodding gratefully.

It isn't long before Tuulik realizes what is happening. As she recovers from her surgery, *The Experiments* shows Macchiarini and the Russian surgeons huddled around her bed in a critical care unit. They are looking at the results of a bronchoscopy, which indicate that the synthetic trachea has folded over. The surgeons seem worried. After some discussion, however, Macchiarini tells Tuulik that the trachea is working perfectly. When she begins to weep, an older Russian surgeon berates her. "Stop crying!" he says. "Remember that the wounds in a winner heal quicker."

Only days after the surgery on Tuulik, Macchiarini tried again with Alexander Zozulya, who, like Tuulik, had a tracheostomy. He died after twenty months.[29] Next came the first child recipient: Hannah Warren, in Peoria, Illinois. Within three months she was dead as well.[30] In January 2014, Andemariam Beyene died. It was the alleged "success" of Beyene's implant that justified the later procedures, yet in *The Experiments*, Macchiarini appears to take the death in stride. On a ferry trip, he meets an old friend and surgical colleague from Turkey, Cengiz Gebitekin, who explains to Lindquist how important it is for a surgeon to be cautious. "The best surgeon knows when not to operate," says Gebitekin, turning to Macchiarini for agreement. Macchiarini does not look up from his phone.

Critical to the success of *The Experiments* is the quiet presence of Lindquist himself. He narrates the documentary in a soft voice, and the first two episodes of *The Experiments* show only glimpses of him, usually in the background of scenes with Macchiarini. When Lindquist finally appears for more extended periods in the final episode, we see a small man with a close-cropped gray beard and a quizzical look on his face. He seems like a kindly, wise philosopher. If anything, Lindquist appears genuinely pained to discover that Macchiarini is a con man and the Karolinska authorities are covering for his crimes.

One of the most eye-opening moments in the film comes when Anders Hamsten, the vice-chancellor of the Karolinska Institute, gives Lindquist an on-camera interview about his decision to exonerate Macchiarini. The contrast between the two men is striking. Blonde and distinguished looking, Hamsten is wearing a dark business suit and a bright yellow tie. Lindquist, modest and unassuming, is dressed in a gray flannel shirt. Yet the impeccably dressed vice-chancellor is incapable of answering the simplest questions. When Lindquist gently presses him to defend the false claims in Macchiarini's *Lancet* paper, Hamsten stammers and professes ignorance with an apologetic smile, as if he expects to be forgiven. If Hamsten had been blustering or arrogant, the interview might be easier to watch. Instead, he just seems bumbling and hapless. It soon becomes clear that the vice-chancellor has personally cleared Macchiarini of wrongdoing in a case about which he knows virtually nothing.

Even more dramatic is the final interview with Macchiarini himself. For the first two episodes of *The Experiments*, Macchiarini appears as a quiet, rather inscrutable presence: self-confident, polite, unruffled by failure. But in the third episode, when Lindquist finally confronts him with hard questions in an interview, he turns contemptuous. He sneers, dodges, and turns Lindquist's questions back on him. "And your profession is?" he asks Lindquist with a self-satisfied smile. "You are a producer, a TV producer, right?" He shrugs. "How can you possibly understand the details of a medical evaluation?" It is as if a disguise has been shed, finally revealing the face beneath the mask.

Public reaction to *The Experiments* was swift. Urban Lendahl, one of Macchiarini's chief defenders, was the first to go. He resigned as secretary-general of the Nobel Assembly in early February. Soon afterward, Anders Hamsten resigned his position as vice-chancellor of the Karolinska Institute.[31] Macchiarini was fired in March. Three months later, he was indicted for manslaughter. In September, after another external review, the Swedish Minister for Higher Education and Research dismissed Harriet Wallberg-Henriksson, chancellor of the Swedish university system, as well as all the remaining members of the board of the Karolinska Institute.[32] Scholars began to question the legitimacy of a Nobel Prize awarded by an institution capable of such deception.[33] For a brief period, it looked as if victory was in sight. But for whistleblowers, of course, victory is never that simple.

· · ·

When I ask Matthias Corbascio if his experience at the Karolinska Institute has changed him, he answers yes without pausing. "I basically have stopped doing research, more or less," he says. The experience opened his eyes not just to Macchiarini's fraud but to the way the entire academic medical system works—how positions are allocated, how hospital administrators make choices, how research funding decisions are made. "It's made me much more cynical," he says. "So, I'm just not going to put my time anymore into doing research. I just lost interest. I'm not interested in research anymore." Like Grinnemo and Simonson, Corbascio has left his position at the Karolinska Institute. Now he works at the Rigshospitalet, in Copenhagen, Denmark, so I am speaking to him by Zoom.

Corbascio grew up in Northern California, the son of an Italian father and a Swedish mother, and he moved to Sweden for his education at Lund University. Even by Zoom, Corbascio projects a slightly intimidating presence, at least at first. He has an intense stare; his head has been shaved bald; and his manner seems guarded, as if he is sizing me up. But as we settle into the conversation, I decide my first impression was mistaken. What initially struck me as severity now seems more like deep moral seriousness. Corbascio listens carefully, and his sense of humor has a dark bitterness that I find familiar. Sometimes disillusionment is so complete that the only reasonable response is to laugh. Corbascio observes his ordeal with a kind of ironic bemusement, as if he is describing a character in a black comedy.

For a time after *The Experiments* aired, the whistleblowers were treated as heroes by the hospital rank and file. But the institutional leaders, including those in the surgical units, still saw them as traitors. "The atmosphere at our department was very, very tyrannical," Corbascio says. He found the atmosphere toxic even before *The Experiments* aired. Once it became clear that the whistleblowers had been right about Macchiarini all along, the departmental leadership ramped up the hostility even more. "They did everything they could subtly to make our existence as painful as possible," Corbascio says. "We'd only get to operate in the afternoon, do the shittiest cases, not develop our skills."

When the head of surgery stepped down in 2016, Corbascio took over as department head—mainly, he says, to protect himself from the former head and his allies. But he found the job unbearable. "Every decision I made as chief of surgery they would question," he says. The criticism was relentless and vicious. "I was investigated twice for malpractice. Both times it turned out I had the best results in the department," he says. Corbascio finally left the Karolinska Institute for his current position in Copenhagen in 2020, four years after Grinnemo and Simonson left for the University of Uppsala.

By no stretch of the imagination could Corbascio be described as a naive idealist. Yet when Corbascio compares what he imagined would happen when Macchiarini was exposed with what actually happened, he marvels at how credulous he was in the beginning. "I was definitely naive, because I thought that when people got to know about this, things would happen. That the university would react," he says. Nor did he anticipate that he and his fellow whistleblowers would be so thoroughly despised after they had been proven right. "It's a question of loyalty, and by doing things that we've done, you have shown yourself to be disloyal to the institution. And disloyalty is worse than lying."

If whistleblower narratives have a consistent theme, it is the ambiguity of their endings. Victory is rare, and never is it uncontested. Even defeat is ambiguous, if only because so many whistleblowers refuse to concede. Sometimes it is possible to identify a resolution to a research scandal after the fact—an official inquiry, a sacrificial firing, a task force—but it usually feels like an artificial construction built to satisfy the demands of a film script or a magazine article. In reality, even successful whistleblowers have a hard time feeling they have won. Once the glare of public attention has faded, most research institutions quietly return to the status quo.

It has been no different at the Karolinska Institute. While two external investigations produced official reports criticizing some aspects of the way the Macchiarini affair was handled, both investigations pointedly avoided the most critical question: How were so many institutional officials able to dismiss credible, documented warnings raised by surgeons with front-row seats for Macchiarini's abuses? Nor did Karolinska leaders take the criticism to heart. When a new vice-chancellor, Ole Petterson, finally conceded in June 2018 that six of Macchiarini's scientific papers were fraudulent and should be retracted, he also announced the astonishing decision to declare three of the whistleblowers guilty as well.[34] Grinnemo was placed in the same category of misconduct as Macchiarini himself, even though he had helped expose the fraud, had taken his name off the *Lancet* paper, and had pressed for years to have the papers retracted.

Yesim Cetir died in March 2017. She underwent an estimated 191 surgical procedures at the Karolinska; by the time of her death she had suffered two strokes, had lost part of her vision, and couldn't walk. Her condition declined significantly in 2013 after Macchiarini's second synthetic implant, but Thomas Fux had managed to keep her alive by developing a custom-made stent with the help of a German company. Her care in the ICU demanded a rigid schedule of bronchoscopies at least every four hours and sometimes as many as fifteen times daily, a brutal regime Simonson compares to water-boarding. In September 2015, Cetir was transferred to Temple University Hospital in Philadelphia for a complex cadaveric transplant, but it failed to save her.[35]

What will happen to Macchiarini is gradually becoming clearer. Eleven of Macchiarini's published papers have been retracted so far, but many others remain in print and are still being cited.[36] In 2018, he published work on the development of an artificial esophagus.[37] In October 2017, Swedish prosecutors dropped the involuntary manslaughter charges against Macchiarini, but in 2020 they reopened the case, instead charging Macchiarini on lesser counts of aggravated assault and severe bodily harm. In June 2022, the court convicted Macchiarini of a single count of "causing bodily harm" to Yesim Cetir and gave him a suspended sentence. But a year later, an appeals court found him guilty of "gross assault" against Andemariam Beyene, Christopher Lyles, and Yesim Cetir and sentenced him to two and a half years in prison. Macchiarini appealed the verdict to Sweden's high court, but in October 2023, his appeal was denied. He has not yet reported to prison.[38]

As Corbascio reflects on the way the Macchiarini case has played out, he tells me a story from his time in high school in California. The police found cocaine in the car of a friend, who proceeded to tell his parents that the cocaine belonged to Corbascio. "So, I was accused of having cocaine," Corbascio says. "I was like, seventeen. I'd never done cocaine. And I remember the feeling of being wrongly accused." The false accusation completely upended his view of how the world worked. He says, "It's sort of the same feeling, where you just feel like there's a total injustice and everything you were taught to believe is shattered."

What destroys such idealistic pictures of the world is not just that offenders go unpunished, but that those who expose the offenses are viewed with such contempt. That comes as a shock to even the most streetwise, cynical whistleblowers. "It's a disillusionment process," Corbascio says. "Your illusions of justice in the world are shaken." Corbascio was raised in an atmosphere of genuine moral commitment. "My parents were just incredibly honest people who would defend the rights of the weak," he says. His mother and father, both immigrants to the United States, were involved in the civil rights movement in San Francisco in the 1960s and '70s. "So, I grew up with that sort of backbone, and then you expect that the rest of the world has some sort of basic moral compass," he says. "And then that gets shattered because you're doing the right thing, but now suddenly, you know, you're basically the equivalent of a pedophile."

Kalle Grinnemo agrees with Corbascio, but he feels that the long battle against the Karolinska has strengthened him. "I'm not afraid of getting complaints from leaders. I know how to act in these situations," Grinnemo says. "They are all educated here in the same schools. I know exactly what they're going to say, how they'll react, how the system works." But the more important reason Grinnemo feels strengthened is a moral one. He lived up to his own ideals. He was threatened, ostracized, and falsely accused, and still he did the right thing. "I have survived, and I know what I've done, and I have done it for the right reason," Grinnemo says. "So, it makes me feel strong."

Not everyone is capable of thinking like this. To hold fast to the conviction that you are doing the right thing when so many others are convinced you are wrong requires an exceptional degree of moral self-confidence. It also demands a willingness to be content with partial victories of the sort that would never satisfy a strict utilitarian. Whistleblowers take a moral gamble that will probably result in bankruptcy. Usually, their only consolation is the moral victory that comes from knowing they have done the right thing in the face of relentless opposition.

For Simonson, moral victory is enough. "There will be so few things in life you can't buy for money. And that's integrity and the reputation that I have gotten. I have proven that I have that integrity," he says. "The most important quality to have is courage. What is true is basically that four people had courage at the Karolinska, out of all these thousands of workers. It's as simple as that. Everybody had a chance to say anything; they didn't. I don't take that personally. I just understand that I am better than them," Simonson says, starting to laugh. "Which is actually true, but it is very obnoxious."

Coming from some people this blunt statement could sound unbearable, but Simonson is so good-humored and sincere that it sounds like an old-fashioned declaration of honor—at least after a few beers at Rolfs Kök. When I tell him this, he replies, "Yeah, yeah, but it is! I feel like that!" Simonson embraces the ethic of honor without a trace of irony. I could be celebrating with Beowulf at the mead hall after his epic battle with Grendel. "For me—and I think my wife loves me for it, but she is also annoyed by it sometimes—this quality, for me, it's very important that I can look myself in the mirror. I don't really care what other people think. But it's very important that I can hold my head up high."

It is not that Simonson doesn't care about the opinions of other people. He is no Thomas Stockmann, making a quixotic declaration of independence. He just doesn't care about the opinions of people he doesn't respect. "For me, that's not important. To be accepted by the wrong people, that's not important to me," he says. "I want to be accepted by myself and by the right people, the people I care about." Among those people are his patients. It is very important to Simonson that his patients know what he did to stop Macchiarini.

Simonson claims he doesn't hold a grudge against anyone involved in the case. But he says it in the way that the winner of a bloody fight might speak of a vanquished opponent who has fought dirty and lost anyway. Then Simonson tells me a story. He and a former Karolinska Institute official still live in the same neighborhood. This official was one of Macchiarini's most important supporters. One day Simonson was shopping in the supermarket with his family when he and the official spotted each other. A second or two passed. Each man acknowledged that he had been seen by the enemy. Then the official turned and fled. "He just put the shopping basket down, and he ran out the door," Simonson says. He pauses for a moment and laughs. Then he says, "That's winning."

Conclusion

It is a cloudy California morning in April of 2017, and I am standing in the lobby of the Richard Nixon Presidential Library and Museum. My father died two months ago, and it feels as if a vast emptiness has opened up beneath my feet. Just why the Nixon Library seemed like a good place to visit I honestly can't say. Maybe it is for the same reason people like to rummage around in the attic of their childhood home. Walking the halls of the Nixon Library is like wandering through a memory palace. Here is a recording of the "smoking gun" tape that implicated Nixon in the Watergate cover-up. Over there is the Colt .45 pistol that Elvis presented to Nixon when he visited the White House in 1970. Watching the grainy footage of Sam Ervin chairing the Senate Watergate hearings is a step into a time capsule that transports me back to the summer of 1973, an Oldsmobile station wagon in the garage and Grand Funk Railroad on the eight-track.

The mystery of human evil is the mystery of human weakness. How did Nixon become so twisted and vindictive? Why did a socially awkward introvert with no talent for public speaking or small talk choose electoral politics as a career? Nixon was intelligent, shrewd, and intellectually curious. His work ethic was second to none; in law school, his nickname was "Iron Butt." He felt a natural empathy for the underdog. As I stand in front of a photo of Nixon as a young congressman, I find myself wondering whether the tragedy of Nixon's life would have unfolded as it did if he had chosen a vocation that did not magnify and reward his character flaws. In electoral politics, people are tempted to lie to the public, break their promises, offer and accept bribes, and flatter those with power and money. To succeed honorably requires an enormous amount of personal integrity and social skill. Nixon had neither. He compensated for his social ineptitude with a ruthless competitiveness, a killer instinct, and a willingness to roll the dice and take big risks. These characteristics propelled him to the very top of a political career that transformed him into a monster.

Like many monsters, Nixon was driven by moral concerns. He justified his grudges and hatreds by convincing himself that his political enemies were destroying the country. His notorious obsession with leaks came out of a genuine conviction that the government insiders who were giving information to the press were guilty of treason. In September 1971, three men sent by Nixon's "plumbers" unit broke into the office of Daniel Ellsberg's psychiatrist in search of information that would discredit Ellsberg, the era's most famous whistleblower. It was a reckless violation of privacy worthy of a police state, yet Nixon never expressed any regrets. "Call it paranoia, but paranoia for peace isn't that bad," he said. "I didn't want to discredit the man as an individual, I couldn't care less about the punk. I wanted to discredit that kind of activity which was despicable and damaging to the national interest."[1]

If, as Paul Begala once said, every White House takes on the personality of the president, then the mystery of Nixon's dark heart is also the mystery of the men who surrounded him. Do corrupt institutions lead people to betray their moral principles, or do they simply change people so much that they no longer have principles to betray? In the Nixon Library collection is a photo of Nixon at his desk in March 1970, surrounded by clean-shaven men with short hair and thin neckties. The atmosphere is one of buttoned-down, masculine competence. By 1973, when all the lies and secrets were coming undone, the White House had become a steaming cauldron of desperation, guilt, and backstabbing paranoia. John Dean had traded his fifths of scotch for half gallons. Jeb Magruder was drinking heavily and needed tranquilizers to sleep. On a trip to Mississippi with the president on Air Force One, John Ehrlichman fantasized about hurling himself between the pilot and the control panel, crashing the plane in a fiery murder-suicide.[2]

As usual, these black thoughts lead me back to my own predicament. "It's not the crime; it's the cover-up that can get you in real trouble," Dean told Nixon, who paid no more attention than the leaders of the University of Minnesota would have. What is remarkable about the way those leaders stonewalled any scrutiny of Dan Markingson's suicide was its breadth and consistency over so many years. By the end, most of those defending the university had nothing whatsoever to do with the study or its oversight. Some had not even been employed at the university when it took place. They had nothing personally to lose from an honest investigation of the study, or from an apology. Yet not a single one of them chose that path. If any of them are tortured by guilt over their role in the scandal, there has been no public indication of it. I'm reminded again of Nixon, who once told his psychiatrist that when he looked in the mirror, it was as if nothing was there.[3]

• • •

It is the convention to end books about whistleblowers with a tribute to their bravery, an affirmation of their necessity, and perhaps a call to arms. Alison Stanger's book *Whistleblowers* ends with a chapter called "Why America Needs Whistleblowers."[4] In *The Whistleblowers: Exposing Corruption in Government and Industry,* Myron and Penina Glazer encourage whistleblowers to see themselves as part of a righteous social movement, unbowed by setbacks and supported by friends and family. Their concluding chapter is called "The Fight Goes On."[5] At the end of *Crisis of Conscience,* Tom Mueller quotes Hannah Arendt on the Reichstag fire: "I was no longer of the opinion that one can simply be a bystander."[6]

While I don't disagree with the sentiments behind these conclusions, I would feel less than fully honest if I simply echoed them. Anyone weighing a decision whether to blow the whistle on abuses to human research subjects needs to understand that whistleblowing is a poor mechanism for institutional reform, and only so much can be done to protect those who speak out. I am the last person to advise anyone to ignore the demands of conscience, but to encourage potential whistleblowers to speak out without noting the long odds of success and the grim personal costs would be like advising them to leap blindfolded off a cliff.

What lies at the bottom? The good news, such as it is, is that the negative consequences of blowing the whistle on abuses to research subjects are not as extreme as they sometimes are in other fields, such as law enforcement, the military, and many areas of government and business. No one in academic medicine really needs to worry about being shot in the face, like Frank Serpico, or about facing a life sentence in prison, as Daniel Ellsberg expected when he leaked the Pentagon Papers. In democratic societies, they will probably not be detained by authorities and forced to sign a retraction, as Dr. Li Wenliang was when he tried to warn his Chinese colleagues of the dangers of SARS-CoV-2.[7] Whistleblowers in medical research may be ostracized, threatened, defamed, demoted, or fired, but their risks are usually nowhere near those taken by, say, dissidents in autocratic political regimes. When these whistleblowers push back on being labeled heroes, it is not false modesty, just a healthy sense of proportion.

Yet it would be equally misleading to understate those risks. Even whistleblowers who are not fired or demoted often come away from their experience deeply scarred, often for reasons they struggle to articulate. They talk about disillusionment, loneliness, and anger, about their struggles with guilt and shame, about a sense of betrayal and crushed idealism. What looks like vindication from the outside rarely feels that way to whistleblowers themselves. Not everyone reacts in the same way, of course. Some whistleblowers walk away from the wreckage unhurt. But nobody should indulge in the fantasy that they will be celebrated for blowing the whistle. It is more likely that they will be vilified, forgotten, or both.

When I began writing this book, I wanted to know whether my experience at the University of Minnesota was unusual. Clearly it was not. None of the physicians I spoke to expressed warm feelings toward the medical institutions that employed them. Many of them had harsh words for the culture of academic medicine more generally: the arrogance, the authoritarianism, the rigid status hierarchy, the soulless anti-intellectualism. It is tempting to conclude that whistleblowing demands a certain degree of alienation from academic medicine, although it is unclear whether the alienation is cause or effect. Either way, there is nothing surprising in their observations. Critics have been saying the same thing for decades. A recent editorial in *The Lancet* decries the "rigid hierarchy and the guru–acolyte model of leadership" in medical research, while a Stanford neurosurgeon writes, "Medicine, much like the military and law enforcement, is still a hierarchical field in which many feel intimidated to speak up."[8]

The comparison to the military and law enforcement is apt, and not just because they all share hierarchical institutional structures. Like soldiers and police officers, physicians are given an extraordinary amount of power over other people. Those who come to physicians for help are often extremely vulnerable by virtue of illness or disability. It is at least partly for this reason that medicine is organized around a moral mission beyond that of a purely business transaction. Otherwise, the potential for abuse would be far too great. In the same way that soldiers might distinguish themselves from mercenaries by virtue of their loyalty to a nation, physicians might distinguish themselves from, say, pharmaceutical company representatives by virtue of their loyalty to their patients. In theory, if not always in practice, the training and acculturation of physicians are governed by a professional ethic.

What sets the stage for disillusionment is the gap between these high-minded professional aspirations and the reality of how academic medical centers react to wrongdoing. When abuses of human subjects come to light, institutional leaders typically cover up the crimes, stonewall the press, protect their researchers, and punish the whistleblowers. Unless they are forced, they do not compensate victims of wrongdoing or apologize to them. Whether academic medical centers are worse in this regard than, say, tobacco companies is not for me to say. But nobody really expects tobacco companies to be guided by a humanitarian mission. Tobacco companies don't raise money with charity drives. Their employees are not honored with "Healthcare Heroes" night at professional sporting events. It is precisely because academic medical centers have traditionally been trusted to serve the public good that oversight of medical research has always been so deferential and forgiving.

The novelist Omar El Akkad has written that it is tempting to think of broken systems mainly as agents of cruelty. A single act of cruelty can resonate for generations, rippling out into fear, anxiety, and an obsession with revenge. Its memory is very difficult to expel. But cruelty is not the main problem with broken systems, writes El Akkad. The weak and the poor are all too capable of cruelty themselves. He writes, "The real engine at the heart of broken systems, the most insidious, burrowing thing, isn't their cruelty: It's the way power obliterates consequences, the certainty that those responsible, by virtue of how deeply the game is rigged in their favor, will always get away with it."[9]

If whistleblowers don't understand at the beginning of their ordeal that the game is rigged, they know it all too well by the end. What begins as a naive belief that others will share their moral outrage often ends in the deflated realization that they never really had a chance. This sense of deflation is usually worse for whistleblowers who hope to right past wrongs. Public exposure might be enough to halt an unethical study, but it is rarely enough to extract an acknowledgment of wrongdoing in the past, much less an apology to the victims or any significant sanctions for the guilty researchers. In fact, those researchers will often be celebrated. The miniature shrine to Eugene Saenger that I saw in the radioisotope laboratory at the University of Cincinnati is not the exception but the rule.

Consider Saul Krugman, the New York University pediatrician who deliberately infected institutionalized, mentally disabled children at the Willowbrook State School with hepatitis A and B. In 1972, the very year that Mike Wilkins helped expose the horrific conditions at Willowbrook and received a photo of his head in a coffin, Krugman's colleagues elected him president of the American Pediatric Society. Eleven years later, Krugman was given the Mary Woodard Lasker Public Service Award. The Lasker Foundation cited his "courageous leadership in conceiving, developing, and testing vaccines against various viral diseases, especially hepatitis B."[10]

Albert Kligman, a renowned dermatologist at the University of Pennsylvania, conducted barbaric experiments on functionally illiterate prison inmates for decades: exposing them to carcinogens, viruses, fungi, and chemical warfare agents; extracting their fingernails and biopsying their internal organs; dosing them with psychedelic drugs for the Department of Defense.[11] Kligman was sanctioned by the FDA for being dishonest about his results. Yet despite it all, he was elected president of the Society for Investigative Dermatology and received honorary doctorates from the University of Utrecht, in the Netherlands, and Heinrich Heine University, in Germany.[12] After his death, the University of Pennsylvania established two chairs and a lectureship in his name.[13]

Chester Southam, the Cornell University oncologist who injected live cancer cells into elderly, nonconsenting patients at the Jewish Chronic Disease Hospital as well as prisoners at the Ohio State Penitentiary, was elected president of the American Association for Cancer Research.[14] John Cutler, who was deeply involved in both the Tuskegee and Guatemala syphilis studies, went on to become acting dean of the School of Public Health at the University of Pittsburgh and was honored with a named lectureship.[15] Robert Heath, for years the head of the Department of Psychiatry and Neurology at Tulane University, performed dubious deep-brain stimulation experiments on vulnerable psychiatric subjects, resulting in at least two deaths and many serious injuries. In the late 1960s, Heath famously attempted to use the same surgical technology to turn a gay patient straight. To this day, Tulane honors his memory with the Robert G. Heath Chair in Psychiatry and Neurology and the Robert G. Heath Lectureship Fund. The alumni group for the Department of Psychiatry and Neurology is named the Robert Heath Society.[16]

Tributes like this are not limited to the scandals of the distant past. During our long battle over psychiatric research abuses at the University of Minnesota, it often felt as if the adversary was not just the university but the entire psychiatric profession. Each new revelation of wrongdoing seemed to result in a professional award to the department chair, Charles Schulz. In 2013, *Schizophrenia Bulletin* gave Schulz the Wayne Fenton Award for Exceptional Clinical Care.[17] A year later, the American College of Psychiatrists gave him the Stanley Dean Award for Research in Schizophrenia.[18] Even his resignation as department chair in 2015 was accompanied by testimonials to his illustrious career.

When an academic medical center honors the researchers responsible for abuses, it sends a message that undermines anything taught in its formal ethics classes. That message is part of what the psychologist Philip Jackson called the "hidden curriculum" of educational institutions: the unofficial, unwritten lessons that stand apart from the formal course of study.[19] The formal ethics course may include the scandals of Tuskegee and Willowbrook, but the hidden curriculum says that the interests of the institution are more important than those of research subjects, that the administration will protect researchers who violate the rules, and that the system is rigged in favor of those with power. It would be hard to come up with a better way to deter potential whistleblowers from speaking out.

• • •

Anyone who tries to blow the whistle on wrongdoing in research on human subjects faces a practical barrier. Who exactly are you supposed to blow the whistle to? In the United States, the natural place to register concerns is the Institutional Review Board (IRB), the primary oversight body charged with protecting subjects. But the IRB answers to institutional authorities. It will have probably approved the study in advance, and it may well know about the problems already. In the seminar on research scandals that I teach, virtually every wrongful research study we examine was given a seal of approval by an IRB or some other internal peer review committee. A whistleblower who goes to the IRB with complaints will usually have no guarantees of confidentiality, and even if the IRB is responsive, it has little formal power apart from the ability to withdraw its approval of a study.

One might imagine that whistleblowers would find support in the field of bioethics. One powerful strand in the bioethics origin myth has it that the field arose in response to abuses of human subjects.[20] Many bioethicists imagine the field as fundamentally opposed to the excesses of medical power and see moral courage as its fundamental professional virtue. In practice, though, bioethics as a field has done little to support whistleblowers. None of the whistleblowers I spoke to viewed bioethicists as their allies, while some felt that bioethicists had been complicit with the enemy. Most saw them in the same way that Humphrey Bogart saw Peter Lorre in *Casablanca*. "You despise me, don't you?" says Lorre, to which Bogart replies, "If I gave you any thought, I probably would."

In theory, some whistleblowers could take their concerns to the federal Office for Human Research Protection (OHRP). In practice, however, the OHRP is a small, ineffective office that no longer does much to respond to complaints.[21] In addition, the jurisdiction of the OHRP is limited to studies funded by the federal government; it will not investigate studies funded by the pharmaceutical or medical device industry. Whistleblowers could try the FDA, but they're likely to be frustrated there as well. The main job of the FDA is drug safety, not the rights and welfare of human subjects. It is poorly equipped to investigate complaints that subjects have been mistreated.

The FDA does not even inform whistleblowers whether it has taken any action on their complaints.

Years ago, when I was giving talks at other universities in order to raise awareness of the Dan Markingson case, I would often be approached afterward by members of the audience. Some of them came with advice. Leaning in close, as if telling me a secret, a man would say, "Here's a tip for you. *60 Minutes*. What you need to do is get this story on *60 Minutes*." Others counseled me to get in touch with a Hollywood director and make a blockbuster feature film. If the audience member happened to belong to a younger demographic, they might advise me to unleash the massive revolutionary power of social media. What I really needed was a viral video, a slogan, and a hashtag.

"Thanks for the suggestion," I'd say. I knew they were well intentioned. But publicizing the issue, especially going to the press, is a harder and more perilous step than many people imagine. To many whistleblowers, making a scandal public is a solution of last resort, like destroying a home to prevent a forest fire from spreading. Once you speak to a journalist, the story is out of your control. Many journalists don't have enough background understanding of medicine or ethics to investigate a story properly. Others, especially science reporters, are too accustomed to cheerleading for the wonders of medical progress to question the motives of researchers. Even the best journalists face pressures that do not serve the interests of whistleblowers. "Every journalist who is not too stupid or full of himself to notice what is going on knows that what he does is morally indefensible," wrote Janet Malcolm. "He is a kind of confidence man, preying on people's vanity, ignorance, or loneliness, gaining their trust and betraying them without remorse."[22]

Whistleblowers willing to go public often struggle to find a reporter who will listen. They don't know what kind of message will get a reporter's attention or which reporters to approach. Sending an anonymous email is unlikely to get a response. Neither is a long, rambling voice message. The problem, of course, is that many whistleblowers are so deep in the hole of paranoia and anger that they're not really in a position to make a cool elevator pitch for their story. They're more like a drowning person, choking and sputtering, frantically grabbing for anything they can find to keep from sinking.

Maybe it is natural for whistleblowers to imagine that the righteousness of their cause will be sufficient to draw others in. The ethical issues just seem so obvious, the injustice so stark. What they often fail to see is the importance of trust. From the outside, it is hard to know if a would-be whistleblower is an honest dissenter or a deranged conspiracy theorist. Some whistleblowers act for self-serving motives. Others play fast and loose with the facts. Many see major crimes where most people would see peccadilloes. Blowing the whistle is often a genuine moral dilemma in which honesty and the public interest must be weighed against competing goods, such as loyalty to close friends or family members. Some violations of the rules do not merit public exposure. Whether you see Linda Tripp as a courageous whistleblower or Judas the Betrayer will depend on whether you believe the public interest was served by her revelations of an intimate affair between Monica Lewinsky and President Clinton.

When I was a graduate student in Scotland in the 1980s, I was part of a medical group that hosted a talk by a celebrated pharmaceutical industry whistleblower named Stanley Adams. A decade earlier, Adams had been jailed by Swiss authorities and held in solitary confinement after he leaked documents showing that his employer, Hoffmann-La Roche, had engaged in price-fixing. The scandal had turned Adams into a cause célèbre in the United Kingdom, and the students at St. Andrews University elected him rector, an honorary position often awarded to political activists and public figures.

When I began writing this book, I thought that Adams would be perfect for an interview. That was before I discovered that in 1994, he had been convicted of hiring a hit man to kill his second wife for the insurance money.[23]

• • •

"Man has a horror of aloneness," Honoré de Balzac wrote. "And of all kinds of aloneness, moral aloneness is the most terrible kind."[24] Over the years, I have been contacted by many solitary whistleblowers, often in the early stages of their struggles. They are searching for something—sympathy, advice, solidarity—and the Internet has led them to me. Some of these people have struck me as utterly broken. They have tried to do the right thing, and the system has responded with crushing brutality. Others are so consumed by the fight that they have lost perspective. They have no interest in talking about strategy, or sharing their feelings, or hearing about the experiences of other whistleblowers. They just want action, preferably by me. Still others seem lost: paralyzed by indecision, uncertain of the way forward, troubled by memories that they can't seem to shake.

Why is blowing the whistle so lonely? To speak out about wrongdoing often is to become radioactive within your institution. Everyone else runs in the opposite direction. Some colleagues will resent whistleblowers or consider them disloyal, while others will be vaguely embarrassed by the disturbance they are creating. But many will simply be frightened of them—not because they believe they are dangerous, but because they're afraid to be seen as fellow travelers. The stigma of the whistleblower is contagious. People distance themselves in the same way they would distance themselves from a patient with a dangerous infectious disease, like Ebola. Even those who secretly sympathize with the whistleblower will often be frightened of admitting it publicly.

Yet the struggle can also change whistleblowers in ways that drive other people away. Not many people can avoid becoming distrustful and demoralized when people they trusted turn against them. Such changes work against whistleblowers in ways they do not see. They become so suspicious of the institution that others think they're paranoid; they appear so enraged that others think they need anger management training; they are so consumed with despair that nobody wants to be in their company. The loneliness of the struggle feeds on itself. The deeper a whistleblower sinks into the hole, the more unpleasant they become; the more unpleasant they become, the less other people want to be around them. Isolation just plunges them deeper into the hole.

"The magic word for whistleblowers is solidarity," says Tom Devine, the legal director of the Government Accountability Project. One of the most dangerous tropes to have emerged around whistleblowing is that of the heroic dissenter, fighting alone against the crowd. Such people exist, and on rare occasions they even succeed. But most of them need the help of others. When institutions are threatened, they inevitably protect themselves by trying to discredit the whistleblower. They will claim that the whistleblower has ulterior motives, or psychiatric problems, or a long history of causing problems in the workplace. These claims are much harder to sustain against a group of whistleblowers standing together. As Devine says, solidarity makes the difference between success and failure.

Solidarity is also critical for psychological protection. Very few of us have the internal resources to fight a long, grueling battle by ourselves. Some people understand this before they blow the whistle, like the four physicians at the Karolinska Institute who banded together to expose the fraud and abuses of Paolo Macchiarini. They may even be part of a loosely organized political movement, like the Fanon Collective on Staten Island or the Junior Faculty Association at the University of

Cincinnati. Yet even those who know what they are up against rarely anticipate just what the ordeal will do to them. They don't know how long it will last or how it will change them. To blow the whistle without allies is dangerous. To do it without the help and support of close friends is like a sentence of indefinite length in solitary confinement.

The act of whistleblowing rests on the faith that exposing a moral outrage will be sufficient to move others to respond, preferably those in positions of authority. In fact, however, exposure is rarely enough. To the limited extent that whistleblowing has succeeded in reforming research on human subjects, it is largely because it has dovetailed with much larger social movements. With the Tuskegee syphilis study, it was the civil rights movement; with the "unfortunate experiment," it was the New Zealand women's movement; with Willowbrook, it was the disability rights movement. But these convergences were more the result of chance than any conscious plan. Most whistleblowers are accidental dissenters, not revolutionaries. They never planned to lead a protest movement. Most of them simply reached a point where they could either speak out or betray something fundamental about themselves, and so they spoke out.

• • •

Why do some people blow the whistle on wrongdoing while others remain silent? It is tempting to speculate that whistleblowers share a common character trait: a readiness to defy orders, a tendency to step out of line, a willingness to break with the group and register their objections. In fact, what whistleblowers share is a common experience. They have responded to wrongdoing in a particular way. It is true that whistleblowing demands dissent, but what leads each person to that place is a complicated mixture of individual character, culture, circumstance, and personal history. For every fiery activist there is a contemplative philosopher; for every stubborn iconoclast there is a courtly gentleman. Some whistleblowers slide into their dissent reluctantly, while others leap into the fire. I am inclined to agree with Tom Mueller, who, after interviewing hundreds of whistleblowers, concludes, "The truth is, there is no whistleblower 'type,' no one personality with unique potential to call out wrongdoing."[25] Anyone could blow the whistle. Or fail to, as the case may be.

If there is a single thread that runs through the stories in this book, it is that whistleblowers act for deeply held moral reasons. Some of them may struggle to explain those reasons. They may even look back on their actions with regret. But none of them acted for reasons that were self-serving, petty, or small-minded. They had nothing to gain by speaking out, and when they faced resistance, they refused to give in. Often, they struggled for years to get some kind of justice for the victims of research abuses, even as that struggle took a vicious toll on their personal lives and their careers. For the most part they did this without much thanks or recognition.

When I listen to their stories, I hear the language of honor. I'm not entirely sure that they all hear it themselves or that it would occur to them to explain their struggles in that way. But most of the fundamental elements of honor are there: courageous resistance, the sense of duty to oneself, the principled code of conduct, and the need not just to do the right thing but to be recognized for it by the people one respects. Of course, it is possible that I hear the ethic of honor so clearly simply by virtue of the fact that I grew up with it—or at least a lapsed Presbyterian, post-Watergate, South Carolina version of honor. It is also true that the echoes of the honor ethic are much easier to hear in some stories than in others. But it is a rare whistleblower's story in which honor is completely absent.

Not everyone will welcome this interpretation. The very

notion of honor strikes some people as objectionable. It feels primitive, reactionary, and violent. When progressives hear the word "honor," they hear a recruiting slogan for the military. Many women see it as part of a moral system in which they are relegated to a role of subservience, their so-called "honor" defended by men. Even worse than honor itself is the related notion that shame has a positive part to play in motivating people to do the right thing. Shame strikes many people as a brutal, belittling way of enforcing social norms that are often arbitrary and unfair. Time and again I have been asked if it might not be better to emphasize human rights or professional ethics rather than a retrograde system of honor.

The problem with that suggestion is that by and large, whistleblowers don't talk about human rights or professional ethics. They talk about their conscience, their self-respect, and their sense of personal integrity. It is true that they rarely invoke the word "honor," but it is not the word itself that is important. The fact that nobody mentions the word "chastity" anymore doesn't mean that the moral norm that it represents has completely vanished. Remnants of the honor ethic are still in our traditions, our language, and our moral emotions. What makes it feel natural to use the language of honor to describe whistleblowing is less about the content of the honor ethic than its structure—in particular, the way that personal integrity has become attached to principled dissent.

That our society has gradually come to accept whistleblowing as an honorable choice represents an ironic twist on the reflexive tendency to see whistleblowers as traitors. The special venom in the word "traitor" comes from the implication that the offending person has acted from self-interest rather than moral principle. As Charles Peters and Taylor Branch write, "The traitor was excoriated as a person without honor of any kind, who, among people willing to die for cause or principle or survival, could shuffle back and forth between opposing camps, sniffing for the highest bidder."[26] Principled whistleblowers reverse that moral calculus. In a corrupt organization driven by money and power, they alone have held onto their ideals.

I don't want to insist on honor or make overblown claims for its importance. I don't believe that the honor ethic is more likely to lead people to choose dissent over loyalty to the group, nor am I trying to argue that we should turn back the clock and restore the honor ethic to its former glory. It would surprise me if people raised in a culture of honor were any more likely to blow the whistle on wrongdoing than those who were not. My point is simply that the honor ethic has not entirely disappeared. If we want to encourage whistleblowing, it helps to understand how honor works.

Take, for example, the primary legal mechanism put in place to encourage whistleblowing at the federal level in the United States: the qui tam lawsuit. These lawsuits encourage people to blow the whistle on fraud and corruption by giving them a share of any money that results from prosecuting the case. From an economic perspective, the idea behind qui tam lawsuits makes perfect sense; surely people are more likely to blow the whistle if they are given a financial incentive. Federal prosecutors are asking people to risk their careers. They can at least try to protect those people from financial devastation.

Yet for whistleblowers who are fundamentally motivated by honor, it is possible that financial incentives might backfire. A financial reward risks turning an act of selflessness into a market transaction. There is a reason why the military rewards heroism with the Congressional Medal of Honor rather than a large financial bonus. Rewarding heroism with money looks a little too much like overtime pay, or maybe a generous tip. (As Michael Walzer writes, "The morality of the bazaar belongs in the bazaar."[27]) Whistleblowers might even be insulted by the implication that they spoke out for financial gain. If honor is in fact the motivation for speaking out, then it might be better to ensure that whistleblowers are also rewarded with formal honors, such as public recognition for honorable behavior.

Or consider the oversight system that is supposed to protect research subjects. It is, quite literally, an honor system. At its very core is the assumption that researchers will follow the rules while no one is looking. No inspectors are standing at the elbow of researchers, checking to make sure that they are not mistreating subjects or depriving them of sound treatment. There is some oversight, of course. Researchers must fill out forms and follow procedures. But for the most part, oversight bodies simply trust researchers to do what they say they will do. The system works like a college honor code; no proctors are present for the exams. If someone cheats, the only way they will be caught is if someone else refuses to let them get away with it.

Yet it is an honor code that looks nothing like one. Medical researchers take no oaths and make no pledges. No ceremonies reinforce the shared values of the research community. There is nothing to suggest the moral seriousness of the research enterprise, no reminder that research subjects may be sacrificing their well-being for the sake of others, just a maze of petty rules and arcane regulations that often have less to do with protecting subjects than with satisfying the demands of a complex bureaucracy. Nobody treats the honor code as a matter of honor, including the functionaries who administer it. It is no wonder that researchers treat research regulations in the same way that they treat the demands of the Internal Revenue Service or the Department of Motor Vehicles.

It seems to be an unfortunate fact that most efforts to blow the whistle on abuses of human subjects fail, at least by the standards of the whistleblowers themselves. I have no empirical studies to prove this claim; in fact, I have a hard time imagining how such a study could be done. But genuine, full-blown success for whistleblowers is hard for me to find. If the moral value of whistleblowing is measured solely by what it has achieved, then the final ledger on blowing the whistle often comes out in the red. It can be hard for whistleblowers to justify actions that have cost them so much and accomplished so little. They need a story in which their sacrifice makes sense.

Yet if the effort to expose wrongdoing is seen as a matter of honor, then success is measured not in material accomplishment but in the achievement of self-respect. And as the political theorist Sharon Krause writes, self-respect depends not on what one gets, but on what one *does*.[28] No one understood this better than Martin Luther King Jr, who used the desire for self-respect to motivate a generation of civil rights activists. King told a powerful story in which the struggle itself was a noble cause, regardless of how the world responded. Simply taking part was a sign of courage, dignity, and principled ambition. Demonstrators couldn't know in advance whether boycotting the Montgomery buses would result in any material gains. Nor could they know whether making themselves unwelcome at a lunch counter in Rock Hill or Greensboro would ever desegregate restaurants. That they took part anyway, at great risk to themselves, is a testament to the moral power that honor carries.

· · ·

Many people remember where they were when Kennedy was shot or when the towers of the World Trade Center collapsed. I remember exactly where I was when I heard that Nixon had resigned. Along with a group of friends and my younger brother, Hal, I had spent the week at a basketball camp near Lancaster, South Carolina. The camp was a self-enclosed bubble: sleeping in cabins, no television, no radio, just eating and breathing basketball. My mother told us the news when she picked us up at the end of the week. Days had passed since Nixon had flashed the two-handed victory sign from his helicopter on the White House lawn, a plastic smile frozen on his face. I can remember riding home in the back seat of the station wagon, feeling kind of dazed. Gerald Ford had told the nation that our long national nightmare was over, and nobody had thought to wake us up. Was this really how such things ended?

Over eight years have passed now since the Office of the Legislative Auditor delivered its verdict on the Dan Markingson case. Sometimes it feels like a lifetime ago; at other times it feels like yesterday. The span of time since then encompasses the election and defeat of Donald Trump, a worldwide coronavirus pandemic, and the killing of George Floyd by Minneapolis police about 2 miles from our house. My father died in 2017 after his third episode of septic shock. My mother died less than three years later. In the summer of 2022, just as I was finishing this book, my brother Hal died of a heart attack, sending me into a tailspin of grief and despair unlike anything I had experienced before. At the University of Minnesota, memories of the Markingson case have faded. Many of the faculty members who protested and pushed for an external investigation have either retired or moved. So have most of the administrators who resisted. For a while I was invited to talk about the case in classes taught by other professors, but those invitations dried up a few years ago. Most of the students in my own classes do not know who Dan Markingson was. I consider it my responsibility to make sure they do.

The last time I saw Mary Weiss was in the summer of 2018. I went to visit her in a Saint Paul nursing home after hearing that Mike Howard, her close friend and live-in caregiver, had been arrested. According to Mary, Howard had gotten access to her banking information and emptied her accounts. A more stunning betrayal would be hard to imagine. To all outward appearances, Howard had been Mary's steadfast ally during her long fight with the University of Minnesota. He had taken care of her for years when she was sick and disabled. Mary had trusted him, and so had I. Yet in March of 2021, he pleaded guilty to theft charges and was sentenced to a year in prison with five years of probation. Several months later I got an email from one of Mary's relatives, telling me that Mary had passed away. There was no funeral ceremony. According to the email, Mary had donated her body to the University of Minnesota.

I didn't imagine things ending like this. Even now, I struggle to make sense of it. Had I ever really understood the story? There seems to be no symmetry to it, no moral to be drawn, no sharp lines between honesty and deception. I can see why so many whistleblowers become paranoid. As Fred Alford writes, whistleblowers find it difficult to live with a story that amounts to nothing more than chronology: this thing happened, then this one, and then another one. They need a story that is meaningful. Paranoia fills that need. In a paranoid world, the plot hangs together. The characters can be understood. The ending of the story is coherent. The world may look as menacing as the view from the Nixon White House, but at least it makes sense.

When I'm alone with my thoughts, I often wonder how my life might have turned out if I had never gotten involved in the case. My Enemies List would be a lot shorter, of course. Maybe my dentist wouldn't ask me whether I grind my teeth at night. But what I wonder about is not the series of events cascading from my choice, but rather the person I have become as a result. Has the experience hardened me and made me cynical? Has it turned me paranoid and suspicious, like Nixon? Maybe the ordeal has buried itself deep into my unconscious and affected me in ways that I can't see. "What does not kill me makes me stronger," said Nietzsche, but it didn't exactly work out that way when he contracted syphilis. Nietzsche had a mental breakdown, a series of strokes, and was demented by the time he died.

I try to remember all the ways I have been blessed. Ina and our children are at the top of the list. Just below them are my brothers and the friends who helped me get through the long ordeal. It must have felt like paying daily visits to an angry man in prison who can talk of nothing but his wrongful conviction. For some of them, like Leigh Turner and Niki Gjere, it was like volunteering to join me in my cell. Every time I get a note or a phone call from someone asking for help with a hopeless cause, I think about my breakfast with Arne Carlson at Perkins in Golden Valley. I remember the students and faculty members who held signs and distributed flyers and wrote editorials demanding action on the case. Many of them were strangers to me, yet there they were, carrying a black coffin into a meeting of the Board of Regents, arguing with the security guards, delivering funeral flowers to the president.

A few years ago, my son Crawford and I went down to Charleston to watch a basketball tournament. Crawford had finished college and was working as a bartender in Minneapolis. One afternoon, in between games, we were walking on Folly Beach when Crawford said, "Have I ever mentioned what a disappointment it was when I discovered what regular adults were like?" When he was little, he said, it had never occurred to him that there might be adults who were not like my friends. He just assumed that all adults were basically thoughtful, grounded people with a sense of humor and a sound moral compass. But as he got older, he started to have conversations with other adults—his teachers, the parents of his friends, his coworkers at the pizza joint where he worked after school. It came as a shock to find out how shallow and immature most of them were. After a pause, Crawford said, "Your friends are a very high standard of human being." He intended this as an expression of disillusionment. But I couldn't help hearing it as a compliment.

Disillusionment is a common theme in whistleblower stories. When I ask whistleblowers if their ordeal has changed them, they often tell a story of innocence and experience. The younger, more naive version of themselves has become harder, wiser, and more jaded. I could tell a version of this story myself. Yet my experience has also left me with something closer to the opposite, a powerful sense of emotion at unexpected acts of kindness. I typically feel it welling to the surface when I witness small, selfless gestures, often those done not out of duty but from purity of heart: a sympathetic remark, an unanticipated note, a tender word. "Cast your bread upon the water and it shall be returned to you," my mother used to say. I get choked up easily these days, often on occasions where a public display of emotion will embarrass me. That didn't happen before.

There was a time when I just assumed that whistleblowing was primarily an issue of moral courage. The relevant question was: If you are a witness to wrongdoing, will you have the courage to speak out? Yet that way of putting the question assumes that when you witness wrongdoing you will recognize it for what it is. Often this is not the case. The mistake is imagining yourself with the same character and the same moral sensibility that you have now, only transported into a different setting. The reality is somewhat different, especially in medicine. A central aim of medical training is to change your sensibility, to transform you into a different person, one who doesn't react to death and illness like a civilian anymore. The danger is not just that you will see other people do horrible things and feel too afraid to speak up, but that you will no longer see what they are doing as horrible. You will think: this is simply the way it is done.

Or perhaps you won't. When my father began practicing medicine in Clover, South Carolina, in the late 1950s, the waiting room of every doctor in the area was segregated: one room marked for whites, another one for Blacks. No one saw this as unusual. Segregated waiting rooms were the norm. Yet when my father opened his office, he made sure it had a single waiting room where everyone sat together. Nobody said a word about it, he told me. His patients accepted it quietly, without acrimony or objection. Exactly why my father was able to see segregated waiting rooms as morally wrong I don't really know. It certainly wasn't part of his South Carolina medical training. Nor was it part of his upbringing. To be honest, he didn't even seem to think his decision was all that significant. He never presented it to my brothers and me as an object lesson or as some sort of moral turning point. It was more like common sense. He just saw the right thing to do and did it.

When my father finally left his last rehabilitation unit in November 2014, he couldn't yet walk. He had worked hard on his physical therapy, but he was an eighty-two-year-old man who had spent weeks on ventilators and six months in medical facilities before he finally made it back home. On the Sunday after Thanksgiving, just a couple of days after his discharge, I convinced him to let me take him and my mother to church. It was the same Presbyterian church my brothers and I grew up in, just across the street from my father's office. Quite a few members of the congregation were his patients. My father got dressed and climbed into a wheelchair. It felt good to see him in a coat and tie again.

We arrived about five minutes late through a disability elevator in the back. The organist had finished playing the prelude. As soon as I wheeled my father into the sanctuary, the minister's jaw dropped, and he stopped speaking. The entire congregation turned their heads and gasped. And then, after a second of silence, the church erupted in applause. It went on for an embarrassingly long time. I told my father afterward that he had performed a miracle: he had gotten Presbyterians to clap in church. I doubt that Jesus himself could have managed to do that.

"One of the most significant facts about us may finally be that we all begin with the natural equipment to live a thousand kinds of lives but end in the end having lived only one," Clifford Geertz says in *The Interpretation of Cultures*.[29] That single life we live helps make us the kind of person we are. That everyone changes over time, often dramatically, is obvious to anyone who has been to a college or high school reunion. We are all shaped by the work that we do, the places we live, and the people we choose to spend our lives with. It could hardly be otherwise. Yet those changes are often invisible to us, not just because they are usually slow and gradual, but because our experience of them is internal and subjective. All we know is that the world looks different to us now.

Everyone asks whistleblowers if they would do it again. This is a question about foreknowledge and wisdom gained. If you knew what would happen when you spoke out, would you still take the risk? Were the results worth the cost? But to answer that question honestly requires an imaginative leap. The answer is not just a cost-benefit calculation. It is a referendum on the person you used to be and the one you have become. You probably wish things had gone better. Maybe if you had made better tactical decisions, you would not have wound up in the hole. But very few people wish they had been the kind of person who could see people mistreated and say nothing about it.

How exactly do you tell when you have emerged from the hole? That question still nags at me. Is it a return to normal sleep patterns? A release from your obsessive thoughts? The ability to stop playing Warren Zevon's "Lawyers, Guns and Money" on a loop as you pace furiously around Lake Calhoun?

Maybe it is when you are able to step back from the hole and analyze its dimensions. You walk around it slowly, trying to figure out how you got trapped. The hole doesn't seem quite as terrifying as it used to. You can measure it and compare it with other holes. You might even find it's possible to joke about it for a change. Perhaps you have finally gotten out of the hole when you can peer down into the blackness and marvel at its vast depth without getting a sense of vertigo.

Acknowledgments

W hen I count my blessings, I start with my wife, Ina, and our children, Crawford, Martha, and Lyle, all of whom suffered through a dark period with a lot more love, understanding, and forgiveness than I did. I feel the same way about my brother Britt, who can make me laugh harder than anyone else on the planet. I don't know how I would have gotten through those years without the Ethicator.

One of the many things that my brother Hal and I shared— apart from a childhood room, many hours on a cement basketball court, and the soul-destroying experience of medical school—was a deep, often self-destructive sense of anger at injustice, especially when that injustice was directed at the powerless. Most of us learn to hold our tongues when our jobs depend on keeping quiet. Hal never seemed to learn that lesson, which is one of the reasons we all loved him so much. I miss him every day.

I owe so many debts of thanks to friends and colleagues who helped in the struggle to have the University of Minnesota investigated that I could not possibly list them all, but I can name a few. Let me start with the core group of dissenters in Minnesota: Leigh Turner, Niki Gjere, and Arne Carlson. Without them, the struggle would have been unbearable. Trudo Lemmens stepped up at a very low point and organized a group letter to the Faculty Senate that eventually proved to be a critical turning point. The senate resolution to investigate was pushed through by a group of senators led by Naomi Scheman, Teri Caraway, Karen-Sue Taussig, David Pellow, and Bill Messing. Bill Gleason and Kirk Allison were rare supporters in the academic health center when support there was almost nonexistent. Matt Lamkin went far beyond the call of duty, not just as a friend and confidant but as a potent public voice. Eden Almasude was our activist-in-chief and a critical source of moral support while she was still a medical student. Students for a Democratic Society helped organize a futile (but deeply satisfying) protest at a Board of Regents meeting. Members of the local chapter of Mind Freedom came to our campus events and made the administration deeply uncomfortable. Judy Stone wrote blog posts for *Scientific American* that helped spread the word well beyond Minnesota.

A number of friends helped me through that ordeal in ways far too varied to describe. I owe special debts to Susan Parry, Adriane Fugh-Berman, Kathryn Montgomery, Francoise Baylis, Ray DeVries, Joe Davis, Nancy Olivieri, Chuck Turchick, Emily Smith Beitiks, Amy Snow Landa, Greg Kaebnick, Jing-Bao Nie, Grant Gillett, Monika Clark-Grill, Maran Wolston, Tom Cannavino, Rick Weinstein, Marcia Angell, John Dawson, Mike Palmieri, David Gems, Jessica Russell, Donal Mosher, David Hottinger, Emma Bedor Hiland, Al Levine, David Benatar, and Solly Benatar.

This book was supported by several generous awards and grants, including a John Simon Guggenheim Foundation Fellowship, a National Endowment for the Humanities Public Scholar Award, the Cary and Ann Maguire Chair in Ethics and American History at the John S. Kluge Center at the Library of Congress, and a resident fellowship at the Rockefeller Foundation Bellagio Center. I am thankful not just for their financial help but for the friendships that emerged, especially at the Kluge Center and the Bellagio Center.

Parts of several chapters have appeared in different

forms in earlier publications. Part of chapter one appeared in the *Atlantic*, part of chapter two appeared in the *American Scholar*, part of chapter six in the *Boston Review*, and part of chapter seven in the *New York Review of Books*.

I am grateful to my agent, Andrew Blauner, whose loyalty, honor, and sense of humor have been a part of my life for over two decades now. I also owe a substantial debt of thanks to my editor, Star Lawrence. It was a conversation with Star several years ago that made me understand the voice that this book demanded, and it was his belief in the manuscript that got it published.

If this book would have been impossible without my friends, it is also true that it would have been impossible without my enemies, especially those in positions of power at the University of Minnesota. I can't bring myself to say thanks, but I want to reassure each of them that they have not been forgotten.

A Note on Sources

Wen the COVID pandemic arrived in March of 2020, quite a few of my plans for interviewing whistleblowers had to be revised. Although I am happy with the way things eventually turned out, I should acknowledge that the prospect of contracting or transmitting a potentially deadly virus tends to add an element of anxiety and discomfort to an interview. I am grateful to all the whistleblowers who opened their lives to me, especially under these circumstances.

I was fortunate to have met or at least made some initial contact with most of the whistleblowers in this book before the pandemic began. That made the in-person interviews easier. In many cases I followed up on the in-person interviews with additional phone calls, Zoom calls, and emails. I was able to spend a fair amount of time with Ron Jones, Mike Wilkins, Martha Stephens, and Bosse Lindquist outside of our formal interviews—in the car, over meals or drinks, taking walks— while with other sources, our time together was more limited. For stylistic reasons, I have sometimes combined the comments my sources made during in-person interviews with the subsequent phone calls and emails. I do not think that this changed the substance of their comments, but in order to be sure, I checked back with these sources afterward.

Two of the whistleblowers I spoke to have written excellent books about their experiences. Martha Stephens published

The Treatment: The Story of Those Who Died in the Cincinnati Radiation Tests with Duke University Press in 2002, and Ron Jones published *Doctors in Denial: The Forgotten Women in the Unfortunate Experiment* with the University of Otago Press in 2017. Others provided me with extensive written material. John Pesando was gracious enough to give me a copy of an unpublished manuscript about his experience at the Hutch. Mike Wilkins brought me four boxes of notes, books, letters, photographs, and videotapes about his experience at Willowbrook and let me keep them as I was writing the book.

The whistleblowers I have profiled in the book are not the only ones I spoke to. Over the years I have been contacted by so many witnesses to medical misconduct that I could not possibly keep track of them all. I also conducted several formal interviews with whistleblowers whose stories do not appear in the book. For a variety of complicated reasons, I decided to narrow the scope of the book to whistleblowers who had exposed research that had directly harmed human subjects, rather than research that was deceptive or fraudulent. Other whistleblowers I excluded for practical reasons, such as the difficulty of traveling during the pandemic, or legal confidentiality agreements, or simply because they were unwilling to speak openly on the record. This doesn't mean that I did not learn from those conversations or that their experiences did not influence what I wrote.

Here are the dates and places for the main interviews that I drew on for this book:

Peter Buxtun: July 20–21, 2016, at his home in San Francisco.
James Jones: October 4, 2016, by phone.
Mike Wilkins: May 17, 2019, at the Bryant Lake Bowl diner
      and my house in Minneapolis; May 18, at my house; May
      19, at the Hard Times Cafe in Minneapolis; October 30,
      2020, at his house in Kansas City.

Bill Bronston: March 8, 2020, at his house in Sacramento, California.

Diana McCourt: February 21, 2020, by phone.

John Pesando: July 10, 2017, at Slate Coffee in Seattle; September 21, 2020, at the Louisa Boren Lookout in Seattle; and September 23, 2020, at the site of the old Fred Hutchinson Cancer Research Center buildings in Seattle.

Rainer Storb: October 16, 2020, by phone.

Paul Martin: October 9, 2020, by phone.

Jim Pesando: October 22, 2020, by phone.

Martha Stephens: June 13, 2017, in Cincinnati for a preliminary meeting at her house and over dinner; June 5, 2018, at her house in Cincinnati and at the University of Cincinnati hospital; June 6, 2018, at her house; February 28, 2020, at her house.

Jerone Stephens: February 29, 2020, at Izzy's Deli in Cincinnati.

Dave Logan: June 6, 2018, at breakfast in Cincinnati.

Ron Jones: January 29–30, 2017, at his house in Auckland for an informal meeting; March 6, 2019, by phone; November 18–20, 2019, at his house in Auckland; March 17, 2020, at his house during a longer stay in Auckland, March 12–26, 2020.

Michael Churchouse: March 18, 2020, at his farm outside Auckland.

Mary Whaley: March 16, 2020, at Ron Jones's house in Auckland.

Karl-Henrik Grinnemo: April 14, 2021, by Zoom; August 9, 2021, at a restaurant in Stockholm.

Oscar Simonson: November 19, 2017, by phone; April 23, 2021, by Zoom; August 10, 2021, at Rolf's Koek restaurant in Stockholm.

Matthias Corbascio: July 23, 2021, by Zoom.

Bosse Lindquist: August 14, 2021, at his house in Stockholm.

"Sasha": February 1, 2019, in person; April 4, 2021, by Zoom.

Notes

INTRODUCTION

1. Jeremy Olson and Paul Tosto, "The Death of Subject 13," *St. Paul Pioneer Press*, May 18, 2008; Paul Tosto and Jeremy Olson, "The Safety Net That Didn't Save Him," *St. Paul Pioneer Press*, May 19, 2008; Jeremy Olson and Paul Tosto, "Suicide Lawsuit Lays Bare a Debate; Critics Say Drug Firms' Payments to Doctors Are Conflict of Interest," *St. Paul Pioneer Press*, May 20, 2008.

2. Maura Lerner, "Jury Convicts Garfinkel of 5 Fraud Counts," *Star Tribune*, August 6, 1993; Joe Rigert and Maura Lerner, "University Kept Silent for Four Years on Research Misconduct by Garfinkel," *Star Tribune*, August 12, 1993.

3. Maura Lerner and Joe Rigert, "Professor Accused of Coercing Hmong into 'U' Drug Study," *Star Tribune*, October 10, 1993.

4. Robert Whitaker, "The Lure of Riches Fuels Testing," *Boston Globe*, November 17, 1998; Robert Whitaker, *Mad in America: Bad Science, Bad Medicine, and the Enduring Mistreatment of the Mentally Ill* (New York: Basic Books, 2002), 270–73.

5. The university later agreed to drop the demand if Mary Weiss gave up her right to appeal the judgment.

6. Duff Wilson, "Drug Maker's Email Released in Seroquel Lawsuit," *New York Times*, February 27, 2009.

7. Maura Lerner and Janet Moore, "Drug-Company Records Put U on the Spot," *Star Tribune*, March 19, 2009.

8. Kurt Vonnegut, "The Shape of Stories" (Lecture, Case Scholars Program, Cleveland, Ohio, February 4, 2004). https://progressivespeaker.com/news/kurt-vonnegut-lecture-at-case-western-reserve-university/.

9. "Investigators: U of M Drug Study Criticism Grows," Fox 9 News (Minneapolis, MN: KMSP, May 19, 2014). https://www.youtube.com/watch?v=MbV96IoPlYw.

10. "Investigators: Nurse Questions Integrity of U of M Drug Researchers," Fox 9 News (Minneapolis, MN: KMSP). https://web.archive.org/web/20160610004220/https://www.fox9.com/fox-9-mn-special-archive/1641101-story#.

11. Arne Carlson, "University of Minnesota's Bloat Must End," *Star Tribune*, April 6, 2013.

12. Association for the Accreditation of Human Research Protection Programs, "An External Review of the Protection of Human Research

323

Participants at the University of Minnesota with Special Attention to
Research with Adults Who May Lack Decision-Making Capacity," External
review (University of Minnesota: Association for the Accreditation of
Human Research Protection Programs, February 23, 2015). https://
drive.google.com/file/d/0Bw3yHuGQzD8CRm56NURpaWJnVGM/
view?resourcekey=0-eqFVfNolJ2NwM-MAxQBV3Q.

13. Association for the Accreditation of Human Research Protection
Programs, 88; Jennifer Couzin-Frankel, "Human Subjects Protections
under Fire at the University of Minnesota," *Science*, March 2, 2015.

14. Susan Perry, "U of M Suspends Enrollment in Psychiatric Drug Trials in the
Wake of Scathing Report on Markingson Case," *MinnPost*, March 20, 2015.

15. James Nobles, "A Clinical Drug Study at the University of Minnesota
Department of Psychiatry: The Dan Markingson Case" (St. Paul, MN:
Office of the Legislative Auditor, March 19, 2015).

16. Maura Lerner, "Kaler Acknowledges U Made Misstatements on Drug
Study," *Star Tribune*, March 28, 2015.

17. Katie Thomas, "A Drug Trial's Frayed Promise," *New York Times*, April 19,
2015; Jeremy Olson, "U Psychiatry Chief Steps Down in Wake of Research
Criticism," *Star Tribune*, April 9, 2015.

18. Jan Dugas, "University of Minnesota Department of Psychiatry
Assessment Report" (Minneapolis, MN: University of Minnesota,
December 31, 2015). https://www.twincities.com/wp-content/
uploads/2016/02/Assessment-Rpt.pdf; Matt Lamkin and Carl Elliott,
"University of Minnesota Research Lapses Show Self-Reform Is Failing,"
Star Tribune, February 8, 2016.

19. C. K. Stead, *My Name Was Judas* (London: Harvill Secker, 2006).

20. Stead, *My Name Was Judas*, 170.

21. Stead, *My Name Was Judas*, 35.

CHAPTER 1: THE HONOR CODE

1. Charles Peters and Taylor Branch, *Blowing the Whistle: Dissent in the
Public Interest* (New York: Praeger Publishers, 1972), 4.

2. Carl Bernstein and Bob Woodward, *All the President's Men* (New York:
Simon and Schuster, 1974).

3. Max Holland, "The Myth of Deep Throat," *Politico*, September 10, 2017.

4. Hunter S. Thompson, "Fear and Loathing at the Watergate," *Rolling Stone*,
September 27, 1973.

5. Nicholas von Hoffman, "Leakage," *New York Review of Books*, November
25, 1976.

6. John W. Dean, *Blind Ambition: The White House Years* (New York: Simon
and Schuster, 1976), 288.

7. Dean, *Blind Ambition*, 224.

8. "Conversations between Alexander P. Butterfield and David Thelen about
the Discovery of the Watergate Tapes," *Journal of American History* 75, no.
4 (1989): 1245–62.

9. "Conversations between Alexander P. Butterfield and David Thelen."

10. C. Fred Alford, *Whistleblowers: Broken Lives and Organizational Power*
(Ithaca, NY: Cornell University Press, 2001), 75.

11. Alford, *Whistleblowers*, 63.

12. Alford, *Whistleblowers*, 78.
13. Kwame Anthony Appiah, *The Honor Code: How Moral Revolutions Happen* (New York: W. W. Norton, 2010), 13.
14. Ralph Waldo Emerson, *The Works of Ralph Waldo Emerson: Fireside Edition*, vol. 6 (New York: New York Public Library, 1909), 203.
15. Peter Berger, "On the Obsolescence of the Concept of Honor," *European Journal of Sociology / Archives Européennes de Sociologie* 11, no. 2 (November 1970): 338–47.
16. United Nations General Assembly, *Universal Declaration of Human Rights: Final Authorized Text* (New York: United Nations, Office of Public Information, 1980).
17. Ludwig Wittgenstein, *Philosophical Investigations*, trans. G. E. M. Anscombe, 3rd ed. (The Macmillan Company, 1973), 8.
18. Noah Shachtman, "Marines Wreck Super Geek's Career," *Wired*, November 19, 2010.
19. Tom Mueller, *Crisis of Conscience: Whistleblowing in an Age of Fraud* (New York: Penguin, 2020), 53.
20. Anthony Cunningham, *Modern Honor: A Philosophical Defense* (New York: Routledge, 2013), 121.
21. John W. Dean, *Lost Honor* (New York: Stratford Press, 1982), 19.
22. Frank J. Barrett and Theodore R. Sarbin, "Honor as a Moral Category: A Historical-Linguistic Analysis," *Theory & Psychology* 18, no. 1 (February 1, 2008): 5–25.
23. Appiah, *The Honor Code*, 17.
24. Alford, *Whistleblowers*, 43.
25. Václav Havel, "The Power of the Powerless," *East European Politics and Societies* 32, no. 2 (2018): 353–408.
26. United States Congress House Committee on Government Reform and Oversight Subcommittee on Human Resources, *Institutional Review Boards, a System in Jeopardy: Hearing Before the Subcommittee on Human Resources of the Committee on Government Reform and Oversight, House of Representatives, One Hundred Fifth Congress, Second Session, June 11, 1998* (US Government Printing Office, 1999), 115.
27. Appiah, *The Honor Code*, 204.
28. Cunningham, *Modern Honor*, 121.
29. Ruth Benedict, *The Chrysanthemum and the Sword: Patterns of Japanese Culture* (New York: New American Library, 1946), 223.
30. *The Most Dangerous Man in America: Daniel Ellsberg and the Pentagon Papers, IMDb*, 2009.
31. Alford, *Whistleblowers*, 73.
32. Bertram Wyatt-Brown, *Southern Honor: Ethics and Behavior in the Old South* (New York: Oxford University Press, 1983), 155.
33. Robert Neil Mathis, "Preston Smith Brooks: The Man and His Image," *South Carolina Historical Magazine* 79, no. 4 (1978): 296–310.
34. "Brooks Attack on Sumner," *The Charlotte Democrat*, June 3, 1856.
35. Ryan P. Brown, *Honor Bound: How a Cultural Ideal Has Shaped the American Psyche* (New York: Oxford University Press, 2016), 27–28.
36. Brown, *Honor Bound*, 25.
37. Richard E. Nisbett and Dov Cohen, *Culture of Honor: The Psychology of Violence in the South* (Boulder, CO: Westview Press, 1996), 42–53.

38. Dov Cohen et al., "Insult, Aggression, and the Southern Culture of Honor: An 'Experimental Ethnography,'" *Journal of Personality and Social Psychology* 70, no. 5 (1996): 945–60.

39. Peter A. French, *The Virtues of Vengeance* (Lawrence, KS: University Press of Kansas, 2001).

40. Charles Portis, *True Grit* (New York: Overlook Press, 2010), 204.

41. A. M. Viens and J. Savulescu, "Introduction to The Olivieri Symposium," *Journal of Medical Ethics* 30, no. 1 (February 1, 2004): 1–7.

42. James Turk, "The Canadian Corporate-Academic Complex," *Academe*, October 29, 2010.

43. Arthur Schafer, "Biomedical Conflicts of Interest: A Defence of the Sequestration Thesis—Learning from the Cases of Nancy Olivieri and David Healy," *Journal of Medical Ethics* 30, no. 1 (February 2004): 8–24.

44. Jon Thompson, Patricia Baird, and Jocelyn Downie, *The Olivieri Report: The Complete Text of the Report of the Independent Inquiry Commissioned by the Canadian Association of University Teachers* (Toronto: James Lorimer and Company, 2001).

45. "The Secrecy Clause," *60 Minutes*, December 19, 1999.

46. Alford, *Whistleblowers*, 119.

47. "Conversations between Alexander P. Butterfield and David Thelen."

48. Appiah, *The Honor Code*, 88.

49. "Conversations between Alexander P. Butterfield and David Thelen."

50. Myron P. Glazer and Penina Migdal Glazer, *The Whistleblowers* (Basic Books, 1989), 19.

51. Mueller, *Crisis of Conscience*, 9.

52. Mueller, *Crisis of Conscience*, 40.

53. Hilde Lindemann Nelson, *Damaged Identities, Narrative Repair* (Ithaca, NY: Cornell University Press, 2001).

54. "Conversations between Alexander P. Butterfield and David Thelen."

55. "Conversations between Alexander P. Butterfield and David Thelen."

CHAPTER 2: TUSKEGEE

1. Susan M. Reverby, *Examining Tuskegee: The Infamous Syphilis Study and Its Legacy* (Chapel Hill, NC: The University of North Carolina Press, 2009).

2. Allan M. Brandt, "Racism and Research: The Case of the Tuskegee Syphilis Study," *Hastings Center Report* 8, no. 6 (1978): 21–29.

3. James H. Jones, *Bad Blood: The Tuskegee Syphilis Experiment*, new and expanded ed. (New York: Free Press, 1993).

4. Reverby, *Examining Tuskegee*.

5. R. A. Vonderlehr et al., "Untreated Syphilis in the Male Negro: A Comparative Study of Treated and Untreated Cases," *Journal of the American Medical Association* 107, no. 11 (September 12, 1936): 856–60; Sidney Olansky et al., "Untreated Syphilis in the Male Negro: X. Twenty Years of Clinical Observation of Untreated Syphilitic and Presumably Nonsyphilitic Groups," *Journal of Chronic Diseases* 4, no. 2 (August 1, 1956): 177–85.

6. Jay Katz, "The Consent Principle of the Nuremberg Code: Its Significance Then and Now," in *The Nazi Doctors and the Nuremberg Code*, ed. George Annas and Michael Grodin (New York: Oxford University Press, 1992), 228.

7. John Arras, "The Jewish Chronic Disease Hospital Case," in *The Oxford Textbook of Clinical Research Ethics*, ed. Ezekiel Emanuel et al. (New York: Oxford University Press, 2008).

8. H. K. Beecher, "Ethics and Clinical Research," *New England Journal of Medicine* 274, no. 24 (June 16, 1966): 1354–60.

9. Maurice Henry Pappworth, *Human Guinea Pigs; Experimentation on Man* (London: Routledge & Kegan Paul, 1967).

10. Geoffrey Edsall, "A Positive Approach to the Problem of Human Experimentation," *Daedalus* 98, no. 2 (1969): 463–79.

11. Laura Jeanine Morris Stark, *Behind Closed Doors: IRBs and the Making of Ethical Research*, Morality and Society Series (Chicago: University of Chicago Press, 2012).

12. David J. Rothman, *Strangers at the Bedside: A History of How Law and Bioethics Transformed Medical Decision Making* (New York: Basic Books, 1991), 89.

13. Hans Jonas, "Philosophical Reflections on Experimenting with Human Subjects," *Daedalus* 98, no. 2 (1969): 89.

14. Susan M. Reverby, ed., *Tuskegee's Truths: Rethinking the Tuskegee Syphilis Study*, Studies in Social Medicine (Chapel Hill, NC: University of North Carolina Press, 2000), 105.

15. Reverby, *Tuskegee's Truths*, 513, 519, 103–4.

16. Reverby, *Tuskegee's Truths*, 458–60.

17. Jean Heller, "Syphilis Victims in U.S. Study Went Untreated for 40 Years," *New York Times*, July 26, 1972.

18. Reverby, *Examining Tuskegee*, 76.

19. Alexander Dyck, Adair Morse, and Luigi Zingales, "Who Blows the Whistle on Corporate Fraud?" *Journal of Finance* 65, no. 6 (2010): 2213–53.

20. S. McDonald and K. Ahern, "The Professional Consequences of Whistleblowing by Nurses," *Journal of Professional Nursing: Official Journal of the American Association of Colleges of Nursing* 16, no. 6 (December 2000): 313–21.

21. Aaron S. Kesselheim, David M. Studdert, and Michelle M. Mello, "Whistle-Blowers' Experiences in Fraud Litigation against Pharmaceutical Companies," *New England Journal of Medicine* 362, no. 19 (May 13, 2010): 1832–39.

22. Janet P. Near et al., "Does Type of Wrongdoing Affect the Whistle-Blowing Process?" *Business Ethics Quarterly* 14, no. 2 (April 2004): 219–42; US Merit Systems Protection Board, *Blowing the Whistle in the Federal Government: A Comparative Analysis of 1980 and 1983 Survey Findings* (Washington, DC: US Government Printing Office, 1984).

23. Piero Bocchiaro, Philip G. Zimbardo, and Paul A. M. Van Lange, "To Defy or Not to Defy: An Experimental Study of the Dynamics of Disobedience and Whistle-Blowing," *Social Influence* 7, no. 1 (January 1, 2012): 35–50.

24. Stanley Milgram, *Obedience to Authority: An Experimental View*, repr. ed. (Harper Perennial Modern Classics, 2009).

25. William A. Gamson, Bruce Fireman, and Steven Rytina, *Encounters with Unjust Authority*, Dorsey Series in Sociology (Homewood, IL: Dorsey Press, 1982).

26. Associated Press, "Ex-Chief Defends Syphilis Project," *New York Times*, July 28, 1972.

27. Megha Satyanarayana, "He Was a Champion of Public Health—But Played a Role in the Horrors of Tuskegee. Should a College Expunge His Name?" *STAT*, April 27, 2018.

28. Torsten Ove, "Presidential Panel Excoriates Former Pitt Dean," *Pittsburgh Post-Gazette*, August 9, 2011.

29. Reverby, *Examining Tuskegee*, 108.

30. Carl Elliott, "Justice for Injured Research Subjects," *New England Journal of Medicine* 367, no. 1 (July 5, 2012): 6–8.

31. Reverby, *Tuskegee's Truths*, 154.

32. Susan M. Reverby, "'Normal Exposure' and Inoculation Syphilis: A PHS 'Tuskegee' Doctor in Guatemala, 1946–1948," *Journal of Policy History* 23, no. 1 (January 2011): 6–28.

33. Presidential Commission for the Study of Bioethical Issues, *"Ethically Impossible" STD Research in Guatemala from 1946 to 1948* (Washington DC: BrainFeed Press, 2011), 50.

CHAPTER 3: WILLOWBROOK

1. H. K. Beecher, "Ethics and Clinical Research," *New England Journal of Medicine* 274, no. 24 (June 16, 1966): 371.

2. *Willowbrook: The Last Great Disgrace*, Documentary, WABC-TV Channel 7, 1972.

3. Harold Schmeck, "Five U.S. Scientists Win 1983 Lasker Award," *New York Times*, November 17, 1983.

4. Harold Schmeck, "Researcher, Target of a Protest, Is Lauded at Physicians' Parley," *New York Times*, April 18, 1972.

5. Sydney A. Halpern, *Dangerous Medicine: The Story behind Human Experiments with Hepatitis* (New Haven: Yale University Press, 2021), 141.

6. David J. Rothman and Sheila M. Rothman, *The Willowbrook Wars* (New York: Harper & Row, 1984), 262–64; R. Ward et al., "Infectious Hepatitis; Studies of Its Natural History and Prevention," *New England Journal of Medicine* 258, no. 9 (February 27, 1958): 407–16; Saul Krugman et al., "Infectious Hepatitis: Studies on the Effect of Gamma Globulin and on the Incidence of Inapparent Infection," *Journal of the American Medical Association* 174, no. 7 (October 15, 1960): 823–30.

7. Joel Howell and Rodney Hayward, "Writing Willowbrook, Reading Willowbrook: The Recounting of a Medical Experiment," in *Useful Bodies: Humans in the Service of Medical Science in the Twentieth Century*, ed. Jordan Goodman, Anthony McElligott, and Lara Marks (Baltimore: Johns Hopkins University Press, 2008), 191.

8. S. Krugman, "The Willowbrook Hepatitis Studies Revisited: Ethical Aspects," *Reviews of Infectious Diseases* 8, no. 1 (February 1986): 157–62.

9. Howell and Hayward, "Writing Willowbrook, Reading Willowbrook."

10. Halpern, *Dangerous Medicine*, 146.

11. S. Krugman, J. P. Giles, and J. Hammond, "Viral Hepatitis, Type B (MS-2 Strain). Studies on Active Immunization," *Journal of the American Medical Association* 217, no. 1 (July 5, 1971): 41–45.

12. Halpern, *Dangerous Medicine*, 125–26.

13. Krugman, "The Willowbrook Hepatitis Studies Revisited."

14. Rothman and Rothman, *The Willowbrook Wars*, 265–66.
15. Morton M. Hunt, "Pilgrim's Progress (I)," *New Yorker*, September 22, 1961; Morton M. Hunt, "Pilgrim's Progress (II)," *The New Yorker*, September 29, 1961.
16. William Pepper, "The Children of Vietnam," *Ramparts*, January 1967, 45–69.
17. Luther J. Carter, "Topeka: Psychiatric Aides Shake Up the Old Order," *Science* 162, no. 3849 (1968): 104–6.
18. Jane Kurtin, "Grim Tale of Willowbrook Death: Child Choking, Nurse on Phone," *Staten Island Advance*, February 3, 1972; Jane Kurtin, "Hammond: 'I Don't Have to Tell You Anything': Willowbrook Head Fires 2 Who Spoke Out," *Staten Island Advance*, January 7, 1972; Jane Kurtin, "Willowbrook Protesters Turn Rally into Bedlam," *Staten Island Advance*, February 12, 1972.
19. Rothman and Rothman, *The Willowbrook Wars*, 17.
20. Yael Halon, "Geraldo Rivera Breaks Down in Tears Recalling Horrific 'Smell, Sound and Sight' of Willowbrook Institution," Fox News, January 28, 2020.
21. Rothman and Rothman, *The Willowbrook Wars*, 46.
22. Don Heckman, "Lennon Concert Slated Aug. 30 in All-Day Fete to Aid Retarded," *New York Times*, August 17, 1972.
23. Rothman and Rothman, *The Willowbrook Wars*, 65.
24. Rothman and Rothman, *The Willowbrook Wars*, 23.
25. Erving Goffman, *Asylums: Essays on the Social Situation of Mental Patients and Other Inmates* (Garden City, NY: Anchor Books, 1961).
26. Goffman, *Asylums*, 7.
27. Anne Collins, *In the Sleep Room* (Toronto: Lester & Orpen Dennys Ltd, 1988).
28. Allen M. Hornblum, *Acres of Skin: Human Experiments at Holmesburg Prison* (London: Routledge, 1999), xx.
29. Goffman, *Asylums*, 43.
30. Jonathan Shay, *Achilles in Vietnam: Combat Trauma and the Undoing of Character* (New York: Atheneum, 1994), 20.
31. Shay, *Achilles in Vietnam*, 117–18.
32. Shay, *Achilles in Vietnam*, 115.
33. Jonathan Shay, "Casualties," *Daedalus* 140, no. 3 (July 1, 2011): 184.
34. Andrew Jameton, *Nursing Practice: The Ethical Issues* (Englewood Cliffs, NJ: Pearson College Div., 1984), 6.
35. Richard Cole, "Woman with Down's Syndrome Gets a Heart-Lung Transplant," AP News, January 23, 1996.
36. Sharon R. Krause, *Liberalism with Honor* (Cambridge, MA: Harvard University Press, 2002), 169–79.
37. Martin Luther King Jr, *Why We Can't Wait* (Beacon Press, 2011), 49.

CHAPTER 4: THE HUTCH

1. Duff Wilson and David Heath, "Uninformed Consent—What Patients at 'The Hutch' Weren't Told about the Experiments in Which They Died," *Seattle Times*, March 11, 2001; Duff Wilson and David Heath, "The Blood-Cancer Experiment—Patients Never Knew the Full Danger

of Trials They Staked Their Lives On," *Seattle Times*, March 11, 2001; Duff Wilson and David Heath, "The Whistleblower—He Saw the Tests as a Violation of 'Trusting, Desperate Human Beings,'" *Seattle Times*, March 12, 2001; Duff Wilson and David Heath, "The Breast Cancer Experiment—With a Year or Two to Live, Woman Joined Test in Which She Was Misled—and Died," *Seattle Times*, March 13, 2001; Duff Wilson and David Heath, "The Financier—He Helped Create the Biotech Boom, and When It Went Bust, so Did He," *Seattle Times*, March 14, 2001; Duff Wilson and David Heath, "No Wonder They Call the Place 'Mother Hutch,'" *Seattle Times*, March 14, 2001; David Heath and Duff Wilson, "System's Serious Flaws Have Led Many to Call for Regulatory Reform," *Seattle Times*, March 15, 2001; David Heath and Duff Wilson, "Prospects for Change—The Hutch Zealously Guards Its Secrets," *Seattle Times*, March 15, 2001; "Research Center Responds to Times Stories," *Seattle Times*, March 12, 2001; "Questions and Answers about 'the Hutch,'" *Seattle Times*, March 25, 2001.

2. David Heath, "Trial to Open in Deaths of Cancer Patients at Hutch," *Seattle Times*, February 1, 2004.

3. Wilson and Heath, "The Blood-Cancer Experiment—Patients Never Knew the Full Danger."

4. Wilson and Heath, "The Blood-Cancer Experiment—Patients Never Knew the Full Danger."

5. Wilson and Heath, "The Blood-Cancer Experiment—Patients Never Knew the Full Danger."

6. Wilson and Heath, "The Blood-Cancer Experiment—Patients Never Knew the Full Danger."

7. Wilson and Heath, "The Blood-Cancer Experiment—Patients Never Knew the Full Danger."

8. Wilson and Heath, "The Blood-Cancer Experiment—Patients Never Knew the Full Danger."

9. Heath, "Trial to Open in Deaths of Cancer Patients at Hutch."

10. Robert Jackall, *Moral Mazes: The World of Corporate Managers*, 20th anniv. ed. (Oxford: Oxford University Press, 2010).

11. Jackall, *Moral Mazes*, 4.

12. Jackall, *Moral Mazes*, 115.

13. Jackall, *Moral Mazes* 116.

14. Jackall, *Moral Mazes*, 73.

15. Jackall, *Moral Mazes*, 72.

16. Grant Fjermedal, *Magic Bullets* (New York: Macmillan, 1984).

17. Fjermedal, *Magic Bullets*, 219.

18. Fjermedal, *Magic Bullets*, 213.

19. Office for the Protection from Research Risks, "Conclusion of Evaluation of Compliance with Assurance M-1008 with Regard to the Complaint Filed by John M. Pesando MD PhD," September 5, 1995; Wilson and Heath, "The Whistleblower—He Saw the Tests as a Violation of 'Trusting, Desperate Human Beings.'"

20. Wilson and Heath, "Uninformed Consent—What Patients at 'The Hutch' Weren't Told."

21. Wilson and Heath, "The Financier—He Helped Create the Biotech Boom."

22. David Heath and Luke Timmerman, "Jury Finds Hutch Not Negligent in 4 Deaths," *Seattle Times*, April 9, 2004.

23. David Heath, "Hutch Witness Sheds Tears over Patient—Efforts Recalled to Curb Protocol That Led to Deaths," *Seattle Times*, February 12, 2004.

24. Heath, "Hutch Witness Sheds Tears."

25. C. Fred Alford, *Whistleblowers: Broken Lives and Organizational Power* (Ithaca, NY: Cornell University Press, 2001), 20.

26. Wilson and Heath, "The Blood-Cancer Experiment—Patients Never Knew the Full Danger."

27. Jackall, *Moral Mazes*, 139.

28. David Heath, "'Hutch' Doctor Tells of Doubts about Experiment—But He Expresses Support for Protocol 126 Colleagues," *Seattle Times*, February 24, 2004.

29. Denise Gellene, "E. Donnall Thomas, Who Advanced Bone Marrow Transplants, Dies at 92," *New York Times*, October 21, 2012.

30. Sheila Kaplan and Shannon Brownlee, "Duke's Hazards: Did Medical Experiments Put Patients Needlessly at Risk?" *US News & World Report* 126, no. 20 (May 24, 1999): 66.

CHAPTER 5: CINCINNATI

1. Eileen Welsome, *The Plutonium Files: America's Secret Medical Experiments in the Cold War* (New York: Dial Press, 1999), 337–51; Martha Stephens, *The Treatment: The Story of Those Who Died in the Cincinnati Radiation Tests* (Durham, NC: Duke University Press, 2002); Gerald Kutcher, *Contested Medicine: Cancer Research and the Military* (Chicago: University of Chicago Press, 2009); David Egilman et al., "A Little Too Much of the Buchenwald Touch? Military Radiation Research at the University of Cincinnati, 1960–1972," *Accountability in Research* 6, no. 1–2 (January 1998): 63–102.

2. "Eugene L. Saenger Fund," University of Cincinnati College of Medicine.

3. Susan M. Reverby, *Examining Tuskegee: The Infamous Syphilis Study and Its Legacy* (Chapel Hill, NC: The University of North Carolina Press, 2009), 190.

4. Stephens, *The Treatment*, 289.

5. *Eugene Saenger Interviewed by Benjamin Felson and Charles Barrett, February, 1984*, Oral History of Medicine in Cincinnati Series (University of Cincinnati Libraries, 1984).

6. Welsome, *The Plutonium Files*, 338.

7. Welsome, *The Plutonium Files*, 338–39.

8. Welsome, *The Plutonium Files*, 341.

9. *Eugene Saenger Interviewed by Benjamin Felson and Charles Barrett, February, 1984.*

10. Stuart Auerbach and Thomas O'Toole, "Pentagon Has Contract to Test Radiation Effect on Humans: Cancer Patients Used in Radiation Testing," *Washington Post*, October 8, 1971.

11. Roger Rapoport, *The Great American Bomb Machine* (New York: Dutton, 1971).

12. Egilman et al., "A Little Too Much of the Buchenwald Touch?" 80–82.

13. Stephens, *The Treatment*, 184–85.

14. Stuart Auerbach, "Faculty Study Hits Whole-Body Radiation Plan," *Washington Post and Times Herald*, January 26, 1972.
15. The Congressional Record—Senate, January 26, 1972, 1359–1361.
16. Letter from Robert W. McConnell MD to US Senator Mike Gravel, January 3, 1972, Congressional Record—Senate, January 19, 1972, 250–254. https://www.congress.gov/92/crecb/1972/01/19/GPO-CRECB -1972-pt1-2-1.pdf; Egilman et al., "A Little Too Much of the Buchenwald Touch?" 94–95; Stephens, *The Treatment*, 315.
17. Egilman et al., "A Little Too Much of the Buchenwald Touch?" 91–93.
18. Kutcher, *Contested Medicine*, 180–83.
19. Stephens, *The Treatment*, 11.
20. Martha Stephens, *Me and the Grandmas of Baghdad* (Cincinnati: PeaceWorks Publishing, 2015), 78.
21. Jerone Stephens, "Political, Social, and Scientific Aspects of Medical Research on Humans," *Politics & Society* 3, no. 4 (1973): 409–35.
22. J. Stephens, "Political, Social, and Scientific Aspects," 417.
23. J. Stephens, "Political, Social, and Scientific Aspects," 429.
24. M. Stephens, *The Treatment*, 17.
25. Eileen Welsome, "The Plutonium Experiment," *Albuquerque Tribune*, November 15, 1993.
26. M. Stephens, *The Treatment*, 17.
27. Nick Miller, "The Secret History of UC's Radiation Tests," *Cincinnati Post*, January 29, 1994.
28. M. Stephens, *The Treatment*, 33.
29. Miller, "The Secret History of UC's Radiation Tests."
30. M. Stephens, *The Treatment*, 21.
31. M. Stephens, *The Treatment*, 22.
32. Martha Stephens, *The Question of Flannery O'Connor*, Southern Literary Studies (Baton Rouge: Louisiana State University Press, 1973), 5.
33. Flannery O'Connor, *The Complete Stories* (New York: Farrar, Straus and Giroux, 1971), 445–82.
34. O'Connor, *The Complete Stories*, 482.
35. Welsome, *The Plutonium Files*, 449.
36. M. Stephens, *The Treatment*, 125.
37. M. Stephens, *The Treatment*, 118–19.
38. Philip J. Hilts, "Panel Urges U.S. to Apologize for Radiation Testing and Pay Damages," *New York Times*, October 3, 1995.
39. Welsome, *The Plutonium Files*, 464.
40. M. Stephens, *The Treatment*, 124.
41. Welsome, *The Plutonium Files*, 463.
42. David Egilman et al., "Ethical Aerobics: ACHRE's Flight from Responsibility," *Accountability in Research* 6, no. 1–2 (January 1998): 15–61.
43. Welsome, *The Plutonium Files*, 468.
44. Welsome, *The Plutonium Files*, 470.
45. Welsome, *The Plutonium Files*, 476.
46. M. Stephens, *The Treatment*, 288.
47. M. Stephens, *The Treatment*, 289.
48. Aaron Lazare, *On Apology* (New York: Oxford University Press, 2005), 52.
49. Lazare, *On Apology*, 39–40.

50. Lazare, *On Apology*, 91.
51. Erving Goffman, *Relations in Public; Microstudies of the Public Order* (New York: Basic Books, 1971), 113.
52. Lazare, *On Apology*, 65.
53. Welsome, *The Plutonium Files*, 469.
54. "Blog Post Leads to Memorial Being Cleaned Up," WCPO 9 Cincinnati, July 3, 2017.

CHAPTER 6: THE UNFORTUNATE EXPERIMENT

1. Sandra Coney and Phillida Bunkle, "An Unfortunate Experiment at National Women's," *Metro*, June 1987.
2. Sandra Coney, *The Unfortunate Experiment*, Penguin Original (Auckland, NZ: Penguin, 1988), 35.
3. Ronald W. Jones, *Doctors in Denial: The Forgotten Women in the "Unfortunate Experiment"* (Dunedin, NZ: University of Otago Press, 2017).
4. Jones, *Doctors in Denial*, 44–45.
5. Coney, *The Unfortunate Experiment*, 56.
6. Jones, *Doctors in Denial*, 46.
7. Jones, *Doctors in Denial*, 18.
8. Coney, *The Unfortunate Experiment*, 51–55.
9. Silvia Cartwright, *The Report of the Committee of Inquiry into Allegations Concerning the Treatment of Cervical Cancer at National Women's Hospital and into Other Related Matters* (Auckland, NZ: The Committee, 1988), 21.
10. H. K. Beecher, "Ethics and Clinical Research," *New England Journal of Medicine* 274, no. 24 (June 16, 1966).
11. Jones, *Doctors in Denial*, 20, 29.
12. Jones, *Doctors in Denial*, 29.
13. Cartwright, *The Report of the Committee*, 21.
14. In 1938, researchers in Boston stopped a study early because the abnormal cells were progressing to cancer. Eighteen years later, a Norwegian study showed that 26 percent of women with CIS had developed cervical cancer within fifteen years. In 1961, a compilation of studies of untreated CIS showed an average of 28 percent of patients developing cancer. In fact, the assumption that CIS progressed to cancer underpinned the adoption of the Pap smear as a screening tool in the 1950s and '60s. See also Cartwright, *The Report of the Committee*, 23–24.
15. Jones, *Doctors in Denial*, 10.
16. Cartwright, *The Report of the Committee*, 26.
17. Cartwright, *The Report of the Committee*, 70–71.
18. Coney, *The Unfortunate Experiment*, 58.
19. Jones, *Doctors in Denial*, 59.
20. Cartwright, *The Report of the Committee*, 21.
21. Coney, *The Unfortunate Experiment*, 61.
22. Jones, *Doctors in Denial*, 82.
23. Jones, *Doctors in Denial*, 76.
24. Jones, *Doctors in Denial*, 72–73.
25. Coney, *The Unfortunate Experiment*, 62–64.
26. Jones, *Doctors in Denial*, 83.

27. Coney, *The Unfortunate Experiment*, 66.
28. Coney, *The Unfortunate Experiment*, 194–95.
29. Coney, *The Unfortunate Experiment*, 69.
30. D. C. Skegg, "Cervical Screening," *New Zealand Medical Journal* 99, no. 794 (January 22, 1986): 26–27.
31. John Knox, *The First Blast of the Trumpet against the Monstrous Regiment of Women*, 1558. Edward Arber, ed. (London: Limited Library Edition, 1880).
32. Bainton, Roland H., and James C. Spalding. "Protestantism—The Role of John Knox." Edited by The Editors of *Encyclopædia Britannica*. *Encyclopædia Britannica*, online ed. https://www.britannica.com/topic/Protestantism/The-role-of-John-Knox.
33. Kristen Walton, *Catholic Queen, Protestant Patriarchy: Mary Queen of Scots and the Politics of Gender and Religion* (London: Palgrave Macmillan, 2006), 97.
34. Donald Macmillan, *John Knox, a Biography* (London: Melrose, 1905), 36, 83, 265.
35. Macmillan, *John Knox, a Biography*, 288.
36. Jones, *Doctors in Denial*, 80.
37. Jones, *Doctors in Denial*, 22.
38. Jones, *Doctors in Denial*, 92–98.
39. Jones, *Doctors in Denial*, 102.
40. W. A. McIndoe et al., "The Invasive Potential of Carcinoma in Situ of the Cervix," *Obstetrics and Gynecology* 64, no. 4 (October 1984): 451–58; Ronald Jones, "The 1984 Article: The Invasive Potential of Carcinoma in Situ of the Cervix," in *The Cartwright Papers: Essays on the Cervical Cancer Inquiry 1987–88* (Wellington, NZ: Bridget Williams Books, 2009).
41. Jones, *Doctors in Denial*, 107.
42. Jones, *Doctors in Denial*, 104.
43. McIndoe et al., "The Invasive Potential of Carcinoma."
44. Coney, *The Unfortunate Experiment*, 11, 17–18.
45. Clare Matheson, *Fate Cries Enough* (Hodder and Stoughton, 1989), 120–22.
46. Matheson, *Fate Cries Enough*, 27–37.
47. Jones, *Doctors in Denial*, 113.
48. Matheson, *Fate Cries Enough*, 65.
49. Matheson, *Fate Cries Enough* 91.
50. Matheson, *Fate Cries Enough*, 122.
51. Coney, *The Unfortunate Experiment*, 41.
52. Coney, *The Unfortunate Experiment*, 41.
53. Coney, *The Unfortunate Experiment*, 41.
54. Coney, *The Unfortunate Experiment*, 73.
55. Coney, *The Unfortunate Experiment*, 76.
56. Joanna Manning, "Report Summary: The Cartwright Report's Findings and Recommendations," in *The Cartwright Papers: Essays on the Cervical Cancer Inquiry 1987–88*, ed. Joanna Manning (Wellington, NZ: Bridget Williams Books, 2009), 28–29.
57. Coney, *The Unfortunate Experiment*, 209.
58. Coney, *The Unfortunate Experiment*, 212.
59. Coney, *The Unfortunate Experiment*, 210.

60. Coney, *The Unfortunate Experiment*, 51–52.
61. Coney, *The Unfortunate Experiment*, 203.
62. Coney, *The Unfortunate Experiment*, 204.
63. Pip Bourke, "Adventure on the High Seas," Stuff, December 22, 2011. https://www.stuff.co.nz/auckland/local-news/eastern-courier/6177280/ Adventure-on-the-high-seas; Michael Churchouse and Judy Churchouse, *Against the Wind* (Michael & Judy Churchouse, 2011).
64. Jones, *Doctors in Denial*, 127.
65. Matheson, *Fate Cries Enough*, 190.
66. "Ethic Guidelines for Research," *New Zealand Herald*, October 15, 1990.
67. Cartwright, *The Report of the Committee*, 75.
68. William Whyte, "Groupthink," *Fortune*, March 1952.
69. Irving L. Janis, *Victims of Groupthink: A Psychological Study of Foreign-Policy Decisions and Fiascoes* (Boston: Houghton Mifflin, 1972), iii.
70. Janis, *Victims of Groupthink*, 3.
71. Jones, *Doctors in Denial*, 18, 33.
72. Jones, *Doctors in Denial*, 184.
73. Albert O. Hirschman, *Exit, Voice, and Loyalty: Responses to Decline in Firms, Organizations, and States* (Cambridge, MA: Harvard University Press, 1970); Elliot Aronson and Judson Mills, "The Effect of Severity of Initiation on Liking for a Group," *Journal of Abnormal and Social Psychology* 59 (1959): 177–81.
74. Cartwright, *The Report of the Committee*, 72.
75. Irving Lester Janis, *Groupthink: Psychological Studies of Policy Decisions and Fiascoes* (Houghton Mifflin, 1983), 257.
76. James C. Thomson, "How Could Vietnam Happen? An Autopsy," *Atlantic*, April 1, 1968.
77. Janis, *Groupthink*, 5.
78. Coney, *The Unfortunate Experiment*, 41.
79. Hirschman, *Exit, Voice, and Loyalty*.
80. J. Little, "Cartwright Report 'Based on a Scam,'" *Dominion Sunday Times*, March 12, 1989.
81. Jan Corbett, "Second Thoughts on the Unfortunate Experiment," *Metro*, July 1990.
82. R. W. Carrell, "Trial by Media," *Notes and Records: The Royal Society Journal of the History of Science* 66, no. 3 (June 2012): 305.
83. Iain Chalmers, "The 'Unfortunate Experiment' That Was Not, and the Indebtedness of Women and Children to Herbert ('Herb') Green (1916–2001)," *Journal of Clinical Epidemiology* 122 (June 2020): A14–20.
84. Linda Bryder, *A History of the "Unfortunate Experiment" at National Women's Hospital* (Auckland, NZ: Auckland University Press, 2009).
85. Bryder, *A History of the "Unfortunate Experiment*," 67–71.
86. Joanne Black, "Finally, the Truth," *New Zealand Listener*, August 14, 2009. https://web.archive.org/web/20200421042949/https://www.noted.co .nz/archive/archive-listener-nz-2009/finally-the-truth.
87. Joanna Manning, ed., *The Cartwright Papers: Essays on the Cervical Cancer Inquiry, 1987–88*, Series 21: Into a New Century (Wellington, NZ: Bridget Williams Books, 2009).
88. Laura Tupou, "Doctors' College Apologises over 'Unfortunate Experiment,'" Radio New Zealand, February 14, 2017.

89. "Auckland District Health Board Apologises for Deadly 'Unfortunate Experiment,' " *New Zealand Herald*, August 26, 2018.

CHAPTER 7: THE KAROLINSKA

1.   *Fatal Experiments: The Downfall of a Supersurgeon*, Documentary, 2016. (The original title in Swedish was *The Experiments*, but it was changed to *Fatal Experiments* when the BBC broadcast an English version. All of my references are to the English version.)
2.   "Woman Given Windpipe Created in Laboratory," CNN.com, November 19, 2008.
3.   Richard Knox, "Cancer Patient Gets First Totally Artificial Windpipe," NPR, July 8, 2011.
4.   Philipp Jungebluth et al., "Tracheobronchial Transplantation with a Stem-Cell-Seeded Bioartificial Nanocomposite: A Proof-of-Concept Study," *Lancet* 378, no. 9808 (December 10, 2011): 1997–2004.
5.   Camilla Turner, " 'Cover-Up' over UCL Stem Cell Deaths as Two Young Women Die after Experimental Treatment," *Telegraph*, October 30, 2018.
6.   Henry Fountain, "Synthetic Windpipe Is Used to Replace Cancerous One," *New York Times*, January 12, 2012.
7.   Andreas De Block, Pierre Delaere, and Kristien Hens, "Philosophy of Science Can Prevent Manslaughter," *Journal of Bioethical Inquiry* 19. no. 4 (2022): 537–543.
8.   David Holmes, "Paolo Macchiarini: Crossing Frontiers," *Lancet* 379, no. 9819 (March 10, 2012): 886.
9.   *A Leap of Faith: A Meredith Vieira Special*, NBC News, June 27, 2014.
10. Matthias Corbascio et al., "Analysis of Clinical Outcome of Synthetic Tracheal Transplantation Compared to Results Published in 6 Articles by Macchiarini et al.," Karolinska Institute, August 2014, 24.
11. Laura Beil, "Dr. Death, Season 3: Miracle Man," Lab Rats, accessed November 4, 2022. https://www.youtube.com/watch?v=RtR8QjPyljY.
12. Beil, "Dr. Death."
13. Corbascio et al., "Analysis of Clinical Outcome of Synthetic Tracheal Transplantation," 14.
14. Corbascio et al., "Analysis of Clinical Outcome of Synthetic Tracheal Transplantation."
15. Niels Lynöe, Ethics Council of Karolinska Institute letter to Vice-Chancellor Anders Hamsten, April 12, 2015. http://retractionwatch.com/wp-content/uploads/2015/04/2445_001.pdf.
16. "The Macchiarini Case: Timeline," News from Karolinska Institute, accessed September 12, 2023. https://news.ki.se/the-macchiarini-case-timeline.
17. Henry Fountain, "Leading Surgeon Is Accused of Misconduct in Experimental Transplant Operations," *New York Times*, November 24, 2014.
18. Eve Herold, "A Star Surgeon Left a Trail of Dead Patients—And His Whistleblowers Were Punished," Leaps.org, October 8, 2018, accessed September 12, 2023. https://leaps.org/a-star-surgeon-left-a-trail-of-dead-patients-and-his-whistleblowers-were-punished/.
19. Bengt Gerdin, Statement of Opinion on Assignment ref. 2-2184/2014, Uppsala, May 13, 2015; Gretchen Vogel, "Karolinska Releases English

Translation of Misconduct Report on Trachea Surgeon," *Science*, May 27, 2015.

20. Henry Fountain, "Regenerative Medicine Researcher Cleared of Scientific Misconduct Charges," *New York Times*, August 28, 2015.

21. "Paolo Macchiarini Is Not Guilty of Scientific Misconduct," *Lancet* 386, no. 9997 (September 5, 2015): 932.

22. Henrik Ibsen, *An Enemy of the People: A Play in Five Acts*, trans. R. Farquharson Sharp (Overland Park, KS: Digireads.com Publishing, 2011), 25.

23. Ibsen, *An Enemy of the People*, 87.

24. Ibsen, *An Enemy of the People*, 87.

25. Ibsen, *An Enemy of the People*, 116.

26. Henrik Berggren and Lars Trägårdh, *The Swedish Theory of Love: Individualism and Social Trust in Modern Sweden* (Seattle: University of Washington Press, 2022), 14.

27. Andrew Brown, "Sweden and the World-Historical Power of Conformity during the Coronavirus Pandemic," *Foreign Policy*, October 5, 2020.

28. Adam Ciralsky, "The Celebrity Surgeon Who Used Love, Money, and the Pope to Scam an NBC News Producer," *Vanity Fair*, January 5, 2016.

29. William Kremer, "Paolo Macchiarini: A Surgeon's Downfall," BBC News, September 10, 2016.

30. Henry Fountain, "Young Girl Given Bioengineered Windpipe Dies," *New York Times*, July 8, 2013.

31. Gretchen Vogel, "Karolinska Institute Vice-Chancellor Resigns in Wake of Macchiarini Scandal," *Science*, February 13, 2016.

32. Gretchen Vogel, "Another Scathing Report Causes More Eminent Heads to Roll in the Macchiarini Scandal," *Science*, September 6, 2016.

33. Andreas Vilhelmsson, "The Home of the Nobel: Who Will Blow the Whistle on Academia?" *ECR Community* (blog), October 18, 2016.

34. Alison McCook, "Karolinska Finds Macchiarini, Six Other Researchers Guilty of Misconduct," *Retraction Watch* (blog), June 25, 2018.

35. Emily Whipp et al., "How a Star Surgeon's Personal and Professional Lives Converged to Expose His Lies," ABC News, February 12, 2021.

36. The website Retraction Watch maintains a database of articles that have been retracted, corrected, or flagged for items of concern. Go to http://retractiondatabase.org/.

37. Matt Warren, "Disgraced Surgeon Is Still Publishing on Stem Cell Therapies," *Science*, April 27, 2018.

38. Gretchen Vogel, "Transplant Surgeon Sentenced to Prison for Failed Stem Cell Treatments," *Science*, June 21, 2023.

CONCLUSION

1. "Excerpts From Interview with Nixon about Domestic Effects of Indochina War," *New York Times*, May 20, 1977.

2. Michael Dobbs, *King Richard: Nixon and Watergate: An American Tragedy* (New York: Knopf Doubleday Publishing Group, 2021), 192, 110, 283.

3. Robert Dallek, *Nixon and Kissinger: Partners in Power* (Harper Collins, 2009), 30.

4. Allison Stanger, *Whistleblowers: Honesty in America from Washington to Trump* (New Haven: Yale University Press, 2019).

5. Myron P. Glazer and Penina Migdal Glazer, *The Whistleblowers: Exposing Corruption in Government and Industry* (New York: Basic Books, 1989).
6. Tom Mueller, *Crisis of Conscience: Whistleblowing in an Age of Fraud* (New York: Penguin, 2020), 536.
7. Jing-Bao Nie and Carl Elliott, "Humiliating Whistle-Blowers: Li Wenliang, the Response to Covid-19, and the Call for a Decent Society," *Journal of Bioethical Inquiry* 17, no. 4 (2020): 543–47.
8. "Power and Bullying in Research," Editorial, *Lancet* 399, no. 10326 (February 19, 2022): 695; Patrick Anderer, "Lessons for Physicians from 'The Bleeding Edge': If You See Something, Say Something," *STAT* (blog), August 14, 2018.
9. Omar El Akkad, "Murder in the Mohalla," *New York Times*, April 1, 2022.
10. Harold Schmeck, "Five U.S. Scientists Win 1983 Lasker Award," *New York Times*, November 17, 1983; Mark Hofschneider, "Vaccines for Hepatitis B and Other Infectious Diseases," Lasker Foundation, accessed May 30, 2023. https://laskerfoundation.org/winners/vaccines-for-hepatitis-b-and-other-infectious-diseases/.
11. Allen M. Hornblum, *Acres of Skin: Human Experiments at Holmesburg Prison* (London: Routledge, 1999).
12. Walter F. Naedele, "Albert M. Kligman, 93, Dermatology Researcher," *Philadelphia Inquirer*, February 21, 2010.
13. Alexander Kafka, "This Researcher Exploited Prisoners, Children, and the Elderly. Why Does Penn Honor Him?" *Chronicle of Higher Education*, November 9, 2019. In 2021, after years of public pressure, Penn Medicine apologized and removed Kligman's name from one of the chairs. See Robert Moran, "Penn Medicine Apologizes for Doctor," *Philadelphia Inquirer*, August 21, 2021.
14. Allen M. Hornblum, "NYC's Forgotten Cancer Scandal," *New York Post*, December 29, 2013.
15. Susan M. Reverby, "Enemy of the People/Enemy of the State: Two Great(ly Infamous) Doctors, Passions, and the Judgment of History," *Bulletin of the History of Medicine* 88, no. 3 (2014): 403–30.
16. Carl Elliott, "Happiness on Demand?" *New York Review of Books*, February 7, 2019.
17. Peter F. Buckley, "2013 Wayne Fenton Award for Exceptional Clinical Care," *Schizophrenia Bulletin* 39, no. 5 (September 1, 2013): 943–44.
18. Sarah Hansen, "Psychiatry Head to Receive Major Award," University of Minnesota Medical School, April 15, 2013. https://med.umn.edu/news-events/medical-school-blog/psychiatry-head-receive-major-award.
19. Philip W. Jackson, *Life in Classrooms*, rev. ed. (New York: Teachers College Press, 1990).
20. Atwood Gaines and Eric Juengst, "Origin Myths in Bioethics: Constructing Sources, Motives and Reason in Bioethic(s)," *Culture, Medicine and Psychiatry* 32 (October 1, 2008): 303–27.
21. Therese Defino, "'Nothing Short of Appalling:' Inaction by HHS Oversight Agencies Sets Off Alarms," *Report on Research Compliance* 14, no. 6 (June 2017): 1–5.
22. Janet Malcolm, *The Journalist and the Murderer*, repr. ed. (New York: Vintage, 1990), 3.

23. Will Bennett, "Whistle-Blower Jailed for Hiring Hitman to Kill Wife," *Independent*, March 15, 1994.
24. Balzac is translated and quoted by Erich Fromm in *Escape from Freedom* (Macmillan, 1994), 18. I came across the quotation in Eyal Press, *Beautiful Souls: Saying No, Breaking Ranks, and Heeding the Voice of Conscience in Dark Times* (New York: Farrar, Straus and Giroux, 2012).
25. Mueller, *Crisis of Conscience*, 535.
26. Charles Peters and Taylor Branch, *Blowing the Whistle: Dissent in the Public Interest* (New York: Praeger, 1972), 288.
27. Michael Walzer, *Spheres of Justice: A Defense Of Pluralism And Equality* (New York: Basic Books, 2008), 109.
28. Sharon R. Krause, *Liberalism with Honor* (Cambridge, MA: Harvard University Press, 2002), 177.
29. Clifford Geertz, *The Interpretation of Cultures: Selected Essays* (New York: Basic Books, 1973), 45.

Index

bitterness felt by, 92
"choiceless choice" made by, 48
common experience of, 301–6
conscience of, 5, 38, 50, 64–65, 86,
    88–89, 127, 163, 210, 217, 245, 290,
    303
conventional view of, 9–10
defeated, 157–63
desire for vengeance in, 56–59
disillusionment of, 32, 280–81, 284,
    291–93, 310
effect of whistleblowing on lives of,
    60–62
ethical obstinacy of, 272
in fiction, 194–99, 268–73
guilt felt by, 26, 30, 51, 83, 116, 121, 211,
    242, 244, 289, 291
as heroes, 5, 27–28, 47–48, 150, 244,
    281, 291, 300, 304
hesitation of, to go to the press, 231
honor of, 18, 42–46, 302–6
idealism of, 61–62, 123, 133–34,
    158–60, 269, 284, 291
lack of institutional support for,
    295–96
loneliness of, 62, 64, 89, 162, 164, 269,
    270, 291, 297, 299–301
loss of respect experienced by, 63
motives of, 36, 37, 49, 56–57, 59, 66,
    298, 300, 303–5
in popular culture, 5
risks taken by, 39, 45, 285
sense of failure felt by, 151
shame felt by, 41, 44–46, 48, 51–53,
    62, 130, 202, 244–45, 303
stories and narratives of, 4–6, 9–10,
    12–13, 19, 21, 23–29, 31–33, 35,
    40, 48, 57, 64–66, 89, 93, 130–32,
    134–35, 157, 163, 170–71, 217, 268,
    282, 302–3, 306, 308, 310
tenacity in, 226
as term, 27, 35–36
Whistleblowers (Stanger), 290
*Whistleblowers: Broken Lives and Orga-
    nizational Power* (Alford), 40–41

*Whistleblowers, The: Exposing Corrup-
    tion in Government and Industry*
    (Glazer and Glazer), 290
Whyte, William
    The Organization Man, 239
Wilkins, Erin, 118
Wilkins, Jody, 95, 130
Wilkins, Mike, 13, 94–100, 104–12, 114,
    116–19, 121–23, 125–31, 293
Willowbrook: The Last Great Disgrace
    (documentary), 96–97, 99, 127–28
Willowbrook hepatitis study, 76, 95–105,
    113, 131, 174, 205, 210, 293, 295, 301
Willowbrook Mile, 205
Willowbrook State School, 13, 76,
    95–102, 104–19, 121–23, 125–29,
    205, 293
Wilson, Duff, 135
"Uninformed Consent," 135–37, 155
Wilson, Sloan, 239
    The Man in the Gray Flannel Suit,
    239
Wired magazine, 43
Wittgenstein, Ludwig, 42–43
Wizard of Oz, The, 13, 35
WKRC, 190, 191–92
women's movement, 301
women's suffrage, 221
Woodward, Bob, 35, 36
    All the President's Men, 36
World Medical Association, 74–75, 95
World Trade Center, 306
World War II, 77, 113, 119, 194, 212, 213
Wretched of the Earth, The (Fanon), 106
Wyatt-Brown, Bertram, 53

X, Malcolm, 110

Yale University, 49, 75, 85–86, 88, 239
Yemen, 237
Yingling, David, 143
Young Lords, 111

Zevon, Warren, 312
Zozulya, Hannah, 278